**Reliability and Long-term Results
of Ceramics in Orthopaedics**

Reliability and Long-term Results of Ceramics in Orthopaedics

4th International CeramTec Symposium March 13, 1999

Laurent Sedel and Gerd Willmann

77 figures
34 tables

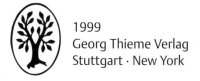

1999
Georg Thieme Verlag
Stuttgart · New York

Die Deutsche Bibliothek – CIP-Einheitsaufnahme
Reliability and long-term results of ceramics in orthopaedics: 4th International CeramTec symposium, March, 1999; 34 tables / Laurent Sedel and Gerd Willmann. – Stuttgart ; New York: Thieme, 1999

Wichtiger Hinweis: Wie jede Wissenschaft ist die Medizin ständigen Entwicklungen unterworfen. Forschung und klinische Erfahrung erweitern unsere Erkenntnisse, insbesondere was Behandlung und medikamentöse Therapie anbelangt. Soweit in diesem Werk eine Dosierung oder eine Applikation erwähnt wird, darf der Leser zwar darauf vertrauen, daß Autoren Herausgeber und Verlag große Sorgfalt darauf verwandt haben, daß diese Angabe **dem Wissensstand bei Fertigstellung des Werkes** entspricht.

Für Angaben über Dosierungsanweisungen und Applikationsformen kann vom Verlag jedoch keine Gewähr übernommen werden. **Jeder Benutzer ist angehalten**, durch sorgfältige Prüfung der Beipackzettel der verwendeten Präparate und gegebenenfalls nach Konsultation eines Spezialisten festzustellen, ob die dort gegebene Empfehlung für Dosierungen oder die Beachtung von Kontraindikationen gegenüber der Angabe in diesem Buch abweicht. Eine solche Prüfung ist besonders wichtig bei selten verwendeten Präparaten oder solchen, die neu auf den Markt gebracht worden sind. **Jede Dosierung oder Applikation erfolgt auf eigene Gefahr des Benutzers.** Autoren und Verlag appellieren an jeden Benutzer, ihm etwa auffallende Ungenauigkeiten dem Verlag mitzuteilen.

© 1999 Georg Thieme Verlag
Rüdigerstraße 14
D – 70469 Stuttgart
(http://www.thieme.de)

Printed in Germany

Umschlaggestaltung:
Martina Berge, Erbach-Ernsbach

Satz: Photocomposition Jung, F-67420 Plaine
Druck: C. Maurer, D-73312 Geislingen/Steige

ISBN 3-13-118481–7   1 2 3 4 5 6

Geschützte Warennamen werden **nicht** besonders kenntlich gemacht. Aus dem Fehlen eines solchen Hinweises kann also nicht geschlossen werden, daß es sich um einen freien Warennamen handele.

Das Werk, einschließlich aller seiner Teile, ist urheberrechtlich geschützt. Jede Verwertung außerhalb der engen Grenzen des Urheberrechtsgesetzes ist ohne Zustimmung des Verlages unzulässig und strafbar. Das gilt insbesondere für Vervielfältigungen, Übersetzungen, Mikroverfilmungen und die Einspeicherung und Verarbeitung in elektronischen Systemen.

Preface 4th Int. CeramTec Symposium

It is a great honour and privilege for me to have been invited as President of the 4th International Symposium on Ceramics organized by CeramTec company in March 1999. This meeting that I did attend once in the past was really of very high scientific level. International participants with different backgrounds surgeons or engineers, from different countries and from different companies clearly expressed the open mind of the organisers. Interdisciplinary discussions were conducted about wear, clinical outcome, sliding properties, biomechanics as well as some legislation problem. Very interesting discussions took place about guidelines regarding revision strategy or how to conciliate materials scientists expertise and surgeons awareness of risk evaluation. All these discussions were of real value and could serve in the future to establish clear guidelines to help surgeons, engineers and lawyers when some problems occur regarding ceramic component fracture, implant retrieval and revision strategy.

We heard experiences from Germany, Italy, Japan, Spain, Belgica, Austria, Australia. They addressed different issues and failures rate were sometimes important. But the overall conclusion were on the success of this alumina on alumina couple that demonstrated low wear, excellent sliding properties and excellent biological tolerance. At revision, there was few macrophagic reactions and it appears that this couple compared very well with metal on PE or with the «come back» metal on metal. More basics research on ceramics characteristics conducted by F. Prud-hommeaux, on simulators studies conducted by J.Fisher, on heat generation conducted by G. Bergmann, and on new materials conducted by A.Toni gave many informations about scientific aspects of the field.

Then alumina on alumina couple is a success in the long term. Safety has to be improved and security control always conducted in order to avoid any problems, breakage, wear. Some issues are still under discussion. They concerned bone adaptation to hardness of ceramics, metal backed or polyethylene backed necessity in order to avoid this elasticity mismatch.

The very fast development of this material proved the validity of the choice made some 30 years ago by people such as Pierre Boutin in France and H. Mittelmeier in Germany, even if some other pioneers such as P. Griss abandoned early this material.

Then a great thank to Doctor Willman, to Doctor Butermilch and the CeramTec company that organised this very interesting high levelled symposium. In the future, we hope that another meeting could be conducting dealing in deep with some aspects already addressed and with some others. This will be undertaken in Stuttgart on Febr. 18 and 19, 2000.

Prof. Dr. L. Sedel (Paris)   May 1999

Preface Proc. 4th Int. CeramTec Symposium 1999

Ceramics in THR offer the option to reduce wear wear debris and to solve the problem of particle induced osteolysis. From the beginnings in the 1970s, the field of ceramics in hip joint replacement surgery has expanded greatly, with far more than 2.5 million ceramic components used worldwide since the beginnings. Right from the beginning the research was always interdisciplinary. I think that one of the most important achievement in bioceramics is the cooperation between material scientists, engineers and surgeons.

The development of joint replacements with ceramics femoral heads and ceramics acetabular components is still ongoing in North America, all over Europe, Australia and Japan. One of the objectives of the CeramTec Symposium is and always will be to compile all the results of clinical and technical research and developments and to share them with surgeons and engineers from all over the world.

Prof. W. Puhl (Ulm, Germany), the President of the previous three symposiums, had proposed that the future presidents should be surgeons from other countries than Germany to underline that the CeramTec Symposiums are really international ones. I am Glad Prof. L. Sedel of Paris had accepted to be the President of the 4th International CeramTec Symposium on RELIABILITY AND LONG-TERM RESULTS OF CERAMICS IN ORTHOPAEDICS which was held in Stuttgart, Germany on March 12 and 13, 1999. Prof. Sedel was assisted by Chairman Prof. Neumann (Magdeburg, Germany), Dr. Toni (Bologna, Italy) and Prof. Stock (Braunschweig, Germany).

It has become a tradition that CeramTec at the occasion of its Symposium awards a prize for outstanding studies with regard to the problems of wear in endoprostheses. This year's price was given to Florence Prudhommeaux for a paper about investigations of retrieved ceramic implants. Members of the 1999 jury had been the four German surgeons Prof. Spranger, Prof. Springorum, Prof. Stock, and Prof. Zichner and me.

My hope is that this 4th proceedings provides a review and an update of ceramics in joint replacement for those who work in the field, both clinically and in research and in development. I would like to thank Prof. Sedel, the speakers and the staff of the publisher Georg Thieme Verlag for their help in the compilation of this work.

I would like to thank CeramTec's staff for all the support, my special thanks to Ms. I. Betsch for the excellent organisation of this symposium.

May 1999   Gerd Willmann, M.S. Ph.D.
Plochingen, Germany

Contents / Inhalt

1 Ceramics in Orthopaedics

1.1 Evolution of Alumina/Alumina implants 2
Laurent Sedel

1.2 Concepts and Designs with Ceramics for Total Hip and Knee Replacement 7
Hironobu Oonishi, Hirokazu Amino, Masaru Ueno, Hiroyuki Yunoki

1.3 The Transcend Alumina Ceramic Hip Articulation System. Surgical Technique – Preliminary Results of 51 cases 29
Marc Goossens

1.4 Long-term Experience with the GSP and Anca Fit System 33
R. Alessandrini, G. Ghidoni, E. Tinelli, G. Giaretta

1.5 From Ceramics to Ceramics. Revisions of THR 35
J. Fenollosa, J. Baeza-Noci, P. Seminario

1.6 Analyse unserer Erfahrungen mit Keramik/Keramik-Hüftendoprothesen der ersten Generation (1974–1978) . . 43
P. Griss, A. Claus und G. Scheller

1.7 6-Jahres-Ergebnisse des Axis-Hüftendoprothesensystems, basierend auf 25 Jahren Erfahrung mit Aluminiumoxydhartgleitpaarungen . . 48
B. Schuhmacher, H. Beck, D. Stock

1.8 The Rationale, Short-term Outcome and Early Complications of a Ceramic Couple in Total Hip Arthroplasty 52
N.R. Bergman, D.A. Young

1.9 Analysis of Wear Debris Particles from Alumina on Alumina Ceramic THA . . . 57
M. Böhler, Y. Mochida, Th.W. Bauer, M. Salzer

2 Reliability – Clinical Aspects

2.1 Ceramic Ball Head Retrieval Data 62
G. Willmann

2.2 CeramTec's Recommendations for Revision when Using BIOLOX®forte Femoral Heads 64
G. Willmann

2.3 Vorgangsweise und Erfahrungen für den Wechsel keramischer Kugelköpfe 67
K. Zweymüller

2.4 Revisionsstrategie nach Bruch oder Verschleiß von Keramikkomponenten 69
P. Griss, A. Claus, G. Scheller

2.5 Revisionsstrategie bei der Verwendung von Keramikköpfen 72
M. Fröhling, L. Zichner, R. Koch

2.6 Revision Strategy for Ceramic Implant Failures 75
L. Sedel

3 Reliability – Technical Aspects

3.1 Wear and Debris Generation in Artificial Hip Joints 78
J. Fisher, E. Ingham, M.H. Stone, B.M. Wroblewski, P.S.M. Barbour, A.A. Besong, J.L. Tipper, J.B. Matthews, P.J. Firkins, A.B. Nevelos, J.E. Nevelos

3.2 New Wear Couples for THR – Simulator Testing 82
A. Toni, S. Affatato

3.3 In-vitro Wear Performance of a Contemporary Alumina : Alumina Bearing Couple Under Anatomically-Relevant Hip Joint Simulation 85
S.K. Taylor

3.4 Friction Induced Temperature Increase of Hip Implants 91
G. Bergmann, F. Graichen, A. Rohlmann

3.5 Wear study in the Alumina-zirconia System 96
C. Kaddick, H.G. Pfaff

3.6 Die Materialpaarung Zirkonoxid/Aluminiumoxid im Hüftgelenk – Eine Fallstudie
The Wear Couple Zirconia/Alumina in THR: A Case Study 102
M.M. Morlock, R. Nassutt, M. Honl, R. Janßen, G. Willmann

4 CeramTec Award 1999

4.1 CeramTec Awards for Studies in the Field of Bioceramics 110

4.2 Analysis of Alumina-Alumina Hip Prostheses Wear Behavior after 10 Years of Implantation 111
F. Prudhommeaux, J. Nevelos, M. Amadouche, C. Doyle, A. Meunier, L. Sedel

5 Important References

5.1 A Bibliography of Published Literature on Bioceramics for THR: 1st Update ... 114
G. Willmann

Speakers / Vortragende

President (Chairmen / Sitzungsleiter)
Prof. Laurent Sedel
Chef du Service de Chirurgie Orthopédique et Traumatologique
Hôpital Lariboisière
Paris
France

Dott. Roberto Alessandrini
Divisione di Ortopedia
Ospedale Civico di Piacenza
Piacenza
Italy

Dr. Neil R. Bergman
Orthopaedic Surgeon
Warringal Medical Centre
Heidelberg
Australia

PD Dr.-Ing. Georg Bergmann
Biomechanik-Labor
Oskar-Helene-Heim
Berlin
Germany

Dr. Maximilian Böhler
Oberarzt
Orthopädisches Spital Speising-Wien
Wien
Austria

Prof. Dr. John Fisher
Professor of Mechanical Engineering
Medical and Biological Engineering
University of Leeds
Department of Mechanical Engineering
Leeds
UK

Dr. Markus Fröhling
Oberarzt
Orthopädische Universitätsklinik und Poliklinik Friedrichsheim Frankfurt a.M.
Frankfurt a.M.-Niederrad
Germany

Prof. Dr. Joaquin Fenollosa Gomez
Hospital Dr. Peset
Valencia
Spain

Dr. Marc Goossens
Orthopaedic Surgeon
Klinick Maria Middelares
Ghent
Belgium

Prof. Dr. med. P. Griss
Leiter der Klinik
Klinikum der Philipps-Universität Marburg,
Marburg
Germany

Dr. C. Kaddick[1]
Endolab
Rosenheim

PD Dr. M. Morlock[1]
Arbeitsbereich Biomechanik
TU Hamburg-Harburg

Prof. Dr. med. H.W. Neumann
(Chairmen / Sitzungsleiter)
Klinikdirektor
Otto-von-Guericke-Universität Magdeburg – Medizinische Fakultät
Magdeburg
Germany

---

[1] kein Vortrag auf dem Symposium

Dr. Hironobu Oonishi
Vice Director Osaka-Minami National Hospital
Department of Orthopaedic Surgery
Osaka
586 Japan

Prof. Dr. Paul-Gerhard Schneider
apl. Professor der Universität Köln, Leiter der Klinik für Orthopädie und Sporttraumatologie
Dreifaltigkeitskrankenhaus
Köln
Germany

Dr. Bernd Schuhmacher
Oberarzt
Orthopädische Klinik
Kliniken Herzogin-Elisabeth Heim
Braunschweig
Germany

Prof. Dr. med. Dietrich Stock
(Chairmen / Sitzungsleiter)
Chefarzt der Orthopädischen Klinik
Kliniken Herzogin-Elisabeth-Heim
Braunschweig
Germany

Scott Taylor
Stryker Osteonics
Allendale, NJ
USA

Dr. Aldo Toni
(Chairmen / Sitzungsleiter)
Istituti Ortopedici Rizzoli
Laboratorio Di Tecnologia Dei Materiali
Bologna
Italy

PD Dr. Gerd Willmann
Director R+D Medical Products Division
CeramTec AG
Plochingen
Germany

Prim. Univ.-Prof. Dr. K. Zweymüller
MA 17 – Orthopädisches Krankenhaus Gersthof
Wien
Austria

1 Ceramics in Orthopaedics

1.1 Evolution of Alumina/Alumina implants

Laurent Sedel

Alumina/alumina couple was first implanted in 1970 by Pierre Boutin (2, 3) in France followed by Mittlemeier in Germany (22, 23).

The initial aim was to reduce wear debris already described by J.Charnley (21) and then to enhance long term results in young people. Since this pioneering period more than 100.000 ceramic on ceramic implants were introduced mostly in Europe. Many papers insisted on fracture risk, early clinical failures, osteolysis (15, 20, 26, 39). But other large experiences were more optimistic (1, 11, 16, 17, 28, 32, 33).

Hard on hard materials had the theoretical advantage of very low wear debris generation and low friction if some technical details are fulfilled. These details concerned the material, its geometry, its fixation system and also its surgical implantation. Alumina ceramic being highly oxidized demonstrated initially a high biocompatibility in bulk or particulate forms (6, 12, 13, 15, 25, 26). Fracture toughness and wear are directly related to the material quality that resumed in high purity, high density, low porosity, low grain size (2 to $3\mu m \pm 1$) (7, 24, 38).

Many different alumina qualities and designs have been implanted in the past. Alumina quality improved over time (36). During the first period from 1970 to 1979 alumina ceramics exhibited low density, high porosity, relatively large grain size up to some tenths of microns (36). Mittlemeier design included cementless screw in ring, cementless stem and large head. It resulted in many early failures not directly related to alumina material but to wrong design and difficult surgery (20, 23, 39). Since the seventies, higher security level has been reached. These incremental improvements are related to material quality, design, and alumina material fixation. Conical sleeving has been used to anchor the head on the stem. Metallic cone technology is very demanding regarding accuracy in cone angle manufacturing and roughness. Some alumina head fracture have been related to poor cone technology. If fracture risk is still of some concern, at worst, its calculated risk could be in the order of one per two thousand for a ten year period. It was in the order of 1 % in the initial phase (7, 10).

Regarding tribological properties alumina on alumina couple did exhibit very low friction coefficient (0,01) after a short period of running in (3, 7, 30). Some manufacturors insisted on the necessity to obtain a low initial clearance in the $30\mu m$ range (3, 30). This was obtained by matching the two components. Improvement in machining processes allows now to obtain unmatched components with this low level of clearance. Wear debris were very difficult to obtain from hip simulators explaining why it was only recently that biological studies compared ceramic debris to other tribological materials (4). Then, clinical studies as well as analysis of retrieved alumina components and biological tissues surrounding failed implants were the only way to understand the wear mechanism and the in vivo behavior of the material.

In vivo wear was measured on retrieved implants by J.M.Dorlot (8, 9), A.Walter (36), Plitz and Griss (26). Their conclusion could be summarized as follow: in a normal situation, when the socket did not tilt before retrieval, the wear was always very low. Linear wear was in the order of 5 to $9\mu m$ per year (8, 9). Biological reactions to wear debris were invetigated by Boehler et al (1) and Lerouge et al (18, 19). The usual reaction is of fibrocytic type with very few macrophages and no giant cells. In some special situations when the prosthesis was loosened for a long time or when there was an impingement between the socket and the stem, alumina debris were found in conjunction with metallic debris. In this case, massive macrophagic reaction leaded to foreign body granuloma (3, 4, 30, 33, 37, 39). We found also that zirconia particles used as cement opacifier was partly involved in the macrophagic response (18, 19). The conclusion was also that, in normal situation,

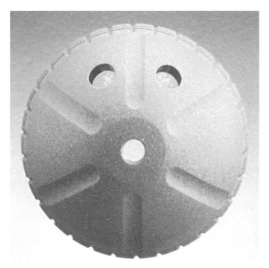

Fig. 1a is the more recent design for the socket: Titanium alloy press-fit cup covered with HA with an alumina liner.

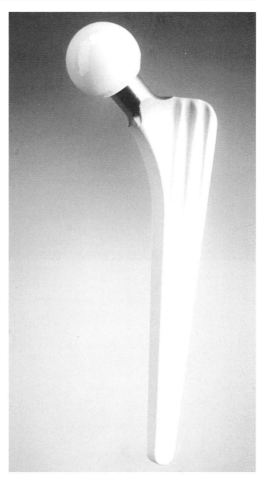

Fig. 1b Cementless stem made of titanium alloy covered with HA with a 32 mm ceramic head manufactured by CERAVER OSTEAL.

debris generation was limited and gave rise to a fibrocytic reaction mainly. In some cases, mechanical loosening was encountered. Mechanical factors and specially alumina rigidity are usually suspected to be responsible for these alumina ceramic loosening (22, 24). In our experience, we suspected poor cement fixation to be the reason for these failures. Regarding the Mittelmeier prosthesis poor, design including the threaded cups was to be blamed. Due to implant mobility, radiolucent lines were described around this prothesis. However, we suspect these radiolucent lines not to be related to a true osteolysis and foreign body reaction even if some papers stated the reverse opinion (38, 39). True foreign body reactions were occasionnaly described by Boutin (3), Boehler (1), ourselves (33) or more recently by Yoon et al (39). They were always related to a very large amount of alumina ceramic debris generated by abnormal contacts (mushroom shaped head, vertical socket) and after a long period of components loosening. Poor alumina quality was also a factor of increased wear as described recently by Prudhommeaux (27). Moreover, to conclude this chapter on biological reaction to alumina debris, the only common conclusion of all clinical papers concerning this sliding couple was the very low rate of osteolysis in all long term series (11, 16, 17, 28, 31, 32, 35). One paper (29) described a sarcoma developped one year after the implantation of a ceramic on ceramic prosthesis. This is the only described case, and one must note that the patient already had a cobalt chromium screw for hip fixation during 15 years.

We started our trial in 1977 with a cemented plain alumina socket and a cemented titanium alloy stem collared, smooth and anodized (24, 31). Clinical results are now available over a twenty years period. Cemented acetabular fixation resulted in an overall 83% survivorship at 10 years and 70% at 15 years. However, results were better in young age population with 86% survivorship at 15 years in patient of less than 50 years of age and the stem depicted a 97% survivorship at 14 years. Most of the revisions were related to the loosening of the cup. Osteolysis was encountered in less than 1% of our cases and was related to patients

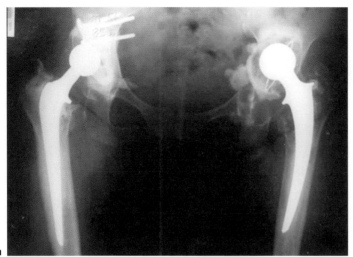

Fig. 2a 37 years old woman had a bilateral total hip implanted 17 years ago. On the left side, she sustained a loosening related to foreign body reaction to polyethylene debris.

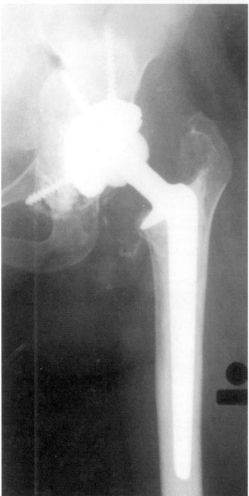

Fig. 2b At revision, we used a reconstruction of the acetabulum with a cementless press-fit socket covered with HA and stabilized by 4 screws. To replace the bone, we used a Biosel* which is a mixture of hydroxyapatite and Beta tri-calcium phosphate and to reconstruct the femoral part, we used a cemented stem. The couple is made of ceramic and ceramic.

with early socket loosening who postponed the revision. These patients demonstrated an impingement problem after the ceramic cup had tilted. The pioneering period (1977-1983) allowed us to document clinical results and to analyze alumina components and tissues retrieved at revision (18, 19, 34). The results confirmed the very low wear rate in vivo: an average of less than 10 µm of linear wear per year was found in normal situations. This value was at least 10 times larger if the prostheses had tilted before revision (8, 9, 27). Histological studies demonstrated the excellent biological tolerance of alumina ceramic debris.

During the last 15 years, we retained the same cemented stem but switched to other means of socket fixation. We limited the use of this material to selected young, active and heavy patients including those having strenuous activities. We tried a screw-in titanium ring with an alumina insert. Some early failures related to this fixation were encountered and, in 1989, a press fit titanium shell with an alumina liner was used. The liner was held by conical sleeving. In selected cases, we also used a plain cementless alumina socket. Survivorship analysis and clinical results on pain and range of motion depicted very similar results to those obtained with more conventional implants. However, roentgenographic studies showed that osteolysis was never encountered while the patients were allowed to perform all type of activities without any limitation.

Results on alumina/alumina allow us to expect an exceptional long term survival in very demanding patients. Fracture risk is now about 1/2000 for a 10 years period (10, 33). As we (and other authors) rarely encounterd osteolysis, any revision becomes a very easy procedure without the need for bone reconstruction. Revision usually concerns the socket and the stem can be left in place. After more than 2000 alumina/alumina couples implanted in our department, we reach the conclusion that this material should be dedicated to young and active people while alumina/polyethylene or metal/polyethylene are still successfull for elderly or less active patients. Providing a good alumina quality, state of the art cone technology and precise surgery, a very long implant survival can be expected. If revision has to be performed, absence of osteolysis results in a surgical situation close to a primary case. Limitation for the use of this material are (i) extra small socket or (ii) the need for small head. We still consider safer to use a 32 mm head diameter even if some teams favor a 28 mm head (apparently without problems).

References

1 Boehler M, Knahr K., Salzer M., Plenk H., Walter A., Schreiber V. Long term results of uncemented alumina acetabular implants. J.bone and Joint Surg. Vol. 76 B, N° 1 January 1994, 53-59.
2 Boutin P., «Arthroplastie Totale de Hanche par Prothèse en Alumine Frittée», Rev.Chir. Orthop. Vol. 58, 1972, pp.229-246.
3 Boutin P., Blanquaert D., «Le Frottement Al/Al en Chirurgie de la Hanche: 1205 Arthroplasties Totales», Rev. Chir. Orthop., Vol. 67, 1981, pp. 279-287.
4 Boutin P., Christel P., Dorlot J.M., Meunier A., de Roquancourt A., Blanquaert D., and al, «The Use of Dense Alumina-Alumina Ceramic Combination in THR», J. Biomat. Mat. Res, V. 22, 1988, p. 1203-1232.
5 Catelas I., Huk O., Petit A., Zukor D.J., Marchand R., Yahia L.H.: Flow cytometric analysis of macrophages mouse response to ceramic and polyethylene particles: effects of size, concentration and composition. J.Biomed.Mater.Res.,41,600-607,1998.
6 Christel P., «Biocompatibility of Surgical-Grade Sense Polycrystalline Alumina», Clin. Orthop. Rel. Res., Vol. 282, 1992, pp.10-18.
7 Clarke I.C. and Willmann G., «Structural Ceramics in Orthopedics», pp. 203-252, In Cameron, ed, Bone Implant Interface, Mosby, 1994.
8 Dorlot J.M., Christel P. and Meunier A., «Wear Analysis of Retrieved Alumina Heads and Sockets of Hip Prostheses», J Biomed. Mater. Res: Applied Biomaterials, Vol. 23, n° A3, 1989 pp.299-310.
9 Dorlot J.M., «Long-Term Effects of Alumina Components in Total Hip Prostheses», Clin. Orthop. Rel. Res, Vol. 282, 1992, pp. 47-52.
10 Fritsch E.W., Gleitz M. Ceramic femoral head fractures in total hip arthroplasty. Clin.Orthop.and Rel. Res. 328,129-136. 1996
11 Garcia-Cimbrelo E., Sayanes J.M., Minuesa A., Munuera L., Mittelmeier Th. «Ceramic-Ceramic Prosthesis after 10 Years», The Journal of Arthroplasty, Vol 11, n° 7, 1996, 773-781.
12 Griss P., Von Andrian-Werburg H., Krempien B. and Heimke G, «Biological Activity and Histocompatibility of Dense Al2O/MgO Ceramic Implants in Rats», J.Biomed.Mater.Res Symp., Vol. 4, 1973 pp. 453-462.
13 Harms J. and Mäusle E., «Tissue Reaction to Ceramic Implant Material», J. Biomed. Mater. Res. Vol. 13, 1979, pp.67-87.
14 Heck D.A., Partridge C.M., Reuben J.D., Lanzer W.L., Lewis C.G., Keating E.M. «Prosthetic Component Failures in Hip Arthroplasty Surgery», The Journal of Arthroplasty, Vol.10, n° 5, 1995, pp.575-580.
15 Heimke G. and Griss P.,» Five Years Experience with Ceramic-Metal-Composite Hip Endoprostheses II. Mechanical Evaluations and Improvements» Arch. Orthop. Trauma. Surgery, Vol. 98, 1981, pp. 165-171.
16 Huo M.H., Martin R.P., Zatorski L.E., Keggi K.J., «Total Hip Replacements Using the Ceramic Mittelmeier

Prosthesis», *Clin.Orthop. and Relat.Res.*, Vol.332, 1996, pp. 143–150.
17. Ivory J.P., Kershaw C.J., Choudry R., Parmar H., Stoyle T.F., «Autophor, Cementless Total Hip Arthroplasty for Osteoarthrosis Secondary to congenital hip dysplasia». *The journal of arthroplasty*, Vol 9, N° 4, 1994, pp. 427–433.
18. Lerouge S., Huk O., Yahia Lh., Witvoet J., Sedel L., «Ceramic-Ceramic vs Metal-Polyethylene: a Comparison of Periprosthetic Tissus from Loosened Total Hip Arthroplasties», *J. Bone and Joint Surg.*, Vol. 79 B,. n° 1, 1997, pp. 135–139.
19. Lerouge S., Huk O., Yahia Lh., Sedel L., «Characterization of in Vivo Wear Debris From Ceramic-Ceramic Total Hip Arthroplasties». *J. of Biom.ed Mat. Res.* Vol.32, 1996, pp. 627–633.
20. Mahoney O.M. and Dimon J.H., «Unsatisfactory Results with a Ceramic Total Hip Prosthesis», *J.Bone Joint Surg.*, Vol. 72A, 1990, pp. 663–671.
21. McKellop H., Clarke I., Markolf K. and Amstutz H., «Friction and Wear Properties of Polymer, Metal and Ceramic Prosthetic Joint Materials Evaluated on a Multichannel Screening Device», *J. Biomed. Mat. Res.*, Vol.15, 1981, pp. 619–653.
22. Meunier A., Nizard R., Bizot P., Sedel L. Clinical Results of Ceramic Bearings in Europe, *Symposium on Alternative Bearing Surfaces in Total Joint Replacement* – ASTM STP *1346*, J.J.Jacobs and T.L. Craig. Eds., American Society for Testing and Materials, 1998.
23. Mittelmeier Th. and Walter A., «The Influence of Prosthesis Design on Wear and Loosening Phenomena», *CRC Critical Reviews in Biocompatibility*, Vol. 3, 1987, pp. 319.
24. Nizard R., Sedel L., Christel P. and al, «Ten-Year Survivorship of Cemented Ceramic-Ceramic Total Hip Prosthesis», *Clin. Orthop. Rel. Res,* Vol. 282, 1992, pp. 53–63.
25. Pizzoferrato A., Cenni E., Ciapetti G., Savarino L. and Stea S., «In Vitro Cytocompatibility and Tissue Reaction to Ceramics», pp.288–291. In: Raviglioli A, Krajewski A., Eds, *Bioceramics and the human body*, Elsevier, The Netherlands, 1992.
26. Plitz W. and Griss P., «Clinical, Histomorphological and Material Related Observations on Removed Alumina-Alumina Hip Joint Components», pp. 131–156, In: Weinstein, Gibbons, Brown & Ruff, Eds, *Implant Retrieval: material and biological analysis*, NBS Special Publication 601, US Dept of Commerce, New York, 1981.
27. Prudhommeaux F., Nevelos J., Doyle C., Meunier A., Sedel L. Analysis of wear behavior of alumina/alumina hip prosthesis after 10 years of implantation. In Bioceramics 11 ;edited by R.Z.Legeros and J.P. Legeros. Proceedings of the 11 International symposium on ceramics in medicine. New York, NY, USA, November 1998. World scientific publishing co, Ptc.Ltd.
28. Riska E.B.Ceramic endoprosthesis in total hip arthroplasty Clin.Orthop 297, 1993, pp.87–94
29. Ryu R.K., Edwin E.G., Skinner H.B. and Murray W.R., «Soft Tissue Sarcoma Associated with Aluminium Oxide Ceramic Total Hip Arthroplasty. A Case Report», *Clin. Orthop. Rel. Res.* Vol. 216, 1987, pp.207–212.
30. Sedel L. «The Tribology of Hip Replacement» *European Instructional Course Lectures*, Edited by Kenwright J., Duparc J., Fulford P., Vol. 3,1997, pp. 25–33.
31. Sedel L., Kerboull L., Christel P., Meunier A., Witvoet J. «Alumina-on-Alumina Hip Replacement: Results and Survivorship in Young Patients», *J. Bone Joint Surg. Vol.72-B, n° 4, 1990, pp. 658–663.*
32. *Sedel L., Nizard R., Kerboull L. and Witvoet J., «Alumina-Alumina Hip Replacement in Patients Younger Than 50 Years Old», Clin.Ortho.Rel.Res. Vol. 298, 1994, pp. 175–183.*
33. Sedel L., Bizot P., Nizard R., Meunier A. Perspective on a 25 years experience with ceramic on ceramic articulation in total hip replacement. Seminars in arthroplasty vol 9, N° 2, 1998,123–134
34. Sedel L., Simeon J., Meunier A., Villette J.M., and Launey S.M., «Prostaglandin E2 Level in Tissue Surrounding Aseptic Failed Total Hips: Effects of Materials», *Arch. Orthop. Trauma. Surg.*, Vol. 111, 1992, pp. 255–258.
35. Toni A., Terzi S., Sudanese A., Tabarroni M., Zappoli F.A., Stea S. Giunti.A., «The Use of Ceramic in Prosthetic Hip Surgery. The State of the Art», *Chir.Organi Mov. LXXX*, 1995, 125–137.
36. Walter A., «On the Material and the Tribology of Al/Al Coupling for Hip Joint Prostheses», *Clin.Orthop. Rel. Res,.* Vol. 282, 1992, pp.31–46.
37. Wirganovicz P.Z., Thomas B.J.,Massive osteolysis after ceramic on ceramic total hip arthroplasty. A case report. Clin.Orthop.N° 338, 1997, 100–104.
38. Wu C., Rice R.W., Johnson D. and Platt B.A., «Grain Size Dependence of Wear in Ceramics», *Ceram. Eng.& Science Proceedings* , Vol. 6, 1985, pp. 995–1011.
39. Taek Rim Yoon, Sung Man Rowe, Sung Taek Jung, Kwang Jin Seon, William, J.Maloney: Osteolysis in association with a total hip arthroplasty with ceramic bearings surfaces. J.Bone and Joint Surg. 80 A , N° 10 Oct. 1998, 1459–1468.

1.2 Concepts and Designs with Ceramics for Total Hip and Knee Replacement

Hironobu Oonishi, Hirokazu Amino, Masaru Ueno, Hiroyuki Yunoki

Introduction

The productions of particulate wear debris from implant materials and subsequent osteolysis has been recognized as the major cause of long term failure in total hip replacement (4, 5, 60, 61, 62). The basic strategy to address the problem of osteolysis should be to reduce the number of polyethylene particles generated by improvement of the materials at the articulating counter faces. The use of a ceramic femoral head has been advocated especially in the young active patients because it produces less polyethylene wear compared with a conventional metal head (8, 51). On the other hand, an attempt to eliminate the use of polyethylene all together has been made through the use of metal on metal and ceramic on ceramic articulations. Although there have also been attempts to improve the wear characteristics of polyethylene, the clinical results have been disappointing, sometimes accompanied by an increased wear rate and osteolysis (1, 7, 59). In our hospital, we used several kinds of socket materials or femoral heads in search of a better articulation in total hip prostheses since 1968 (Fig. 1). In 1970, in order to increase the wear resistance of polyethylene, we performed wear tests on high-density polyethylene (HDP molecular weight was less than one-tenth of UHMWPE) irradiated at several levels of high dose gamma radiation emitted by ^{60}Co. The wear rate was smallest at 100 Mrad (29, 50). Sockets cross-linked by gamma radiation at 100 Mrad were used clinically from 1971 to 1978 (29, 50). As the gamma Radiation Company became bankrupt, these sockets were not used after 1979.

We also experimentally confirmed that ultra high molecular weight polyethylene (UHMWPE)

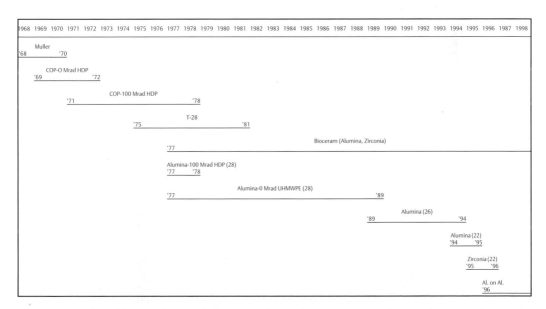

Fig. 1 History of total hip prostheses, which were used in Osaka-Minami National Hospital since 1968 to 1998

showed less wear in an alumina-to-UHMWPE combination than in a metal-to-UHMWPE combination (12, 24). In 1977, we began to use 28 mm-alumina balls. COP alloy (stainless steel containing 20% cobalt) was used for the stem. The prosthesis was named Bioceram. For the socket non-irradiated UHMWPE was used except for 12 cases in which irradiated sockets with 100 Mrad were used. Concurrently we also used the T-28 (stainless steel) stem from Zimmer 1975 to 1981.

From 1977 to 1987, the average grain size of an alumina was 5.6 μm. A ball size was 28 mm. In order to use thicker PE socket, requirement for smaller femoral heads led not only to improvements in alumina quality but also to development of high mechanical strength zirconia. High quality new alumina of 1.4 μm grain size has been used since 1987. Zirconia balls have been used since 1989. Alumina on alumina THP was used since 1996. Bending strength of an alumina, made by Kyocera since 1987, is 650 MPa. Almost grain sizes are less than 2 μm. An average size is 1.4 μm. Experimentally, the bending strength of zirconia aged at 37°C in water for 50 years is forecasted to be more than 1,000 MPa. This value is more than two times higher than ASTM standard for alumina.

In case of ceramic ball fracture after surgery, foreign substances were recognized on the taper surface of the fragments of fractured ceramic ball. Left figure shows a cement thin film of 50 μm in thickness. On the surface tool mark was observed, which was transcribed from the metal taper cone. Right figure was calcium-phosphate thin film (Figure 2). Foreign substances were recognized as bone, soft tissue and bone cement by element analysis (Table 1).

Table 1 Foreign substances were observed by element analysis.

	Element	Material
Case 1	Ca P	Bone
Case 2	Ca C Cl S	Tissue
Case 3	S Ba Cl	Cement

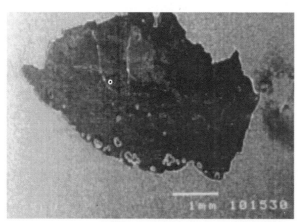
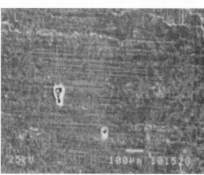
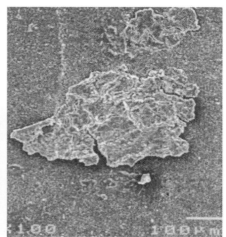

Fig. 2 The foreign substances recognized on the taper surface of the fragments of fractured ceramic ball

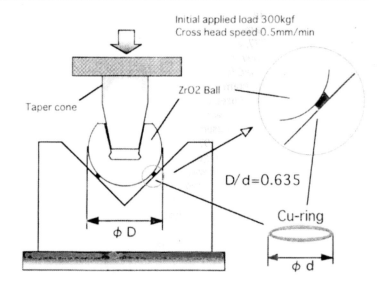

Fig. 3 Ultimate compression strength test model

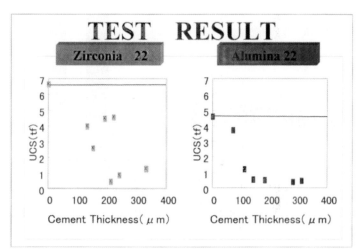

Fig. 4 Ultimate compression strength test result

In order to determine the effect of entrapped foreign substances in the gap between male and female taper, thin bone cement film of 2 X 2 mm rectangular and 70 to 330 μm thickness was entrapped between Ti alloy cone and 22 mm alumina or zirconia balls, and ultimate compression strength test was performed (Figure 3). The average mechanical strength of 22 mm alumina and zirconia ball was 4.66 and 6.66 ton, respectively. After entrapping of foreign substance, mechanical strength decreased less than 10% in both alumina and zirconia ball. Consequently, the taper cone surface must be kept free from foreign bodies (Figure 4). Table 2 is incidence of ceramic ball fracture after surgery in Japan. Before 1990, ball fracture occurred in 0.065% in 28 mm ball, and in 0.036% in 26 mm ball. After 1990, no fracture occurred even in 22 mm ball. Because every surgeon has taken care of entrapping no foreign substance. Fortunately, no fracture in over 3,500 cases occurred in our hospital.

We developed new alumina on alumina THP with polyethylene backed high-quality alumina bearing surface cup and an alumina ball, which was used clinically since 1996. The opening rim of the cup is covered with polyethylene to prevent from alumina-metal neck contact and impingement. In order to determine the optimum design

Table 2 Incidence of ceramic ball fracture after surgery in Japan.

Material: Alumina Ceramics

Size	Period	Cases	Ball-FX (#)	Ball-FX (%)
∅ 22	1990.11 – 1997.2	5,256	0	0.000%
∅ 26	1987.6 – 1997.2	11,551	4	0.036%
∅ 28	1987.12 – 1997.2	3,177	2	0.065%
Total	1987.6 – 1997.2	19,984	6	0.031%

Ball-FX = Ball Fracture

Material: Zirconia Ceramics

Size	Period	Cases	Ball-FX (#)	Ball-FX (%)
∅ 22	1989.2 – 1997.2	1,484	0	0.000%
∅ 26	1996.3 – 1997.2	149	0	0.000%
Total	1989.2 – 1997.2	1,633	0	0.000%

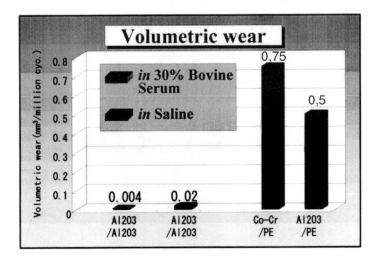

Fig. 5 Volumetric wears of total hip prostheses in hip simulator test

of the bearing surface, we carried out the ultimate compressive strength test and hip simulator wear tests. As a result, sphericity deviation was fixed at ± 1 µm with a radius clearance of 5 to 30 µm. The average grain size of alumina is 1.4 µm and surface finish was controlled to a roughness of less than 0.02 µm. There was no significant difference in fracture load among three different radius clearance ranges of 5–10, 15–20 and 25–30 µm. Wear rate was extremely low and there was no significant difference wear rate among three different clearances (Figure 5).

In our clinical experience, we found that the thicker the polyethylene sockets the lower the wear rate. In order to use a thicker UHMWPE socket the femoral head size was decreased little by little; 26 mm-alumina from 1989 to 1994, 22 mm-alumina from 1994 to 1995, and 22 mm-Zirconia from 1995 to 1996. Since 1996, an alumina on alumina total hip prosthesis have been used because we found the wear of an alumina on alumina total hip prosthesis was extremely low as measured by a hip simulator test (0.004 mm^3/10^6 cycles) (Figure 1). As to ceramic total hip prostheses, in our hospital from 1977 to 1998, about 3,000 alumina balls on UHMWPE sockets, about 350 zirconia balls on UHMWPE sockets, and about 300 alumina on alumina total hip prostheses have been used.

In this study, we measured decreases in the thickness of the socket in vivo to search for a better articulation in total hip prosthesis. In the clinical experience of total hip prostheses with 28-mm alumina heads against UHMWPE sockets since 1977, the decrease in the thickness of the socket against the alumina head was an average of 0.08 mm/year, while that against the metal heads was 0.3 mm/year. Both experimental and clinical results indicated that the wear of the UHMWPE was significantly lower in the combination with alumina than with metal. These advantages led to the development of the alumina total knee prosthesis (KOM).

A combination of alumina and UHMWPE in the sliding portions was used. To determine the mean resistance of alumina total knee prosthesis, knee simulator tests were performed. The simulator test results showed that the decrease in the thickness of the UHMWPE in combination with alumina was less than one-tenth that of the combination with metal (9–19, 34–38, 43–58). An alumina ceramic TKP has been used clinically since January 1982.

[I] Alumina Total Hip Prosthesis

Materials

1) Comparisons of the wear of several kinds of total hip prostheses in our clinical experiences

Decreases in the thickness of the socket (i.e., Wear including creep deformation) of the following five kinds of the total hip prostheses which had been used in our hospital were measured on the radiographs with a refinement of the method of *Levermore* (6).

(1) 100 Mrad irradiated HDP socket with COP alloy head (28 mm)

Polyethylene sockets (High molecular weight polyethylene, Hoechst, Germany, Molecular weight ; 1,000,000) with an inner diameter of 28 mm were irradiated with 100 Mrad gamma radiation in a multiply sealed plastic bag. No special attempt was made to eliminate the ambient air in the plastic bag. During irradiation, the sockets changed color to brown. The femoral components used were a mono block stem made of stainless steel containing 20% cobalt (COP alloy) with a 28 mm head (Out of roundness > 10 μm, Surface roughness > 0.5 μm; Mizuho Medical Instruments Company Ltd. Japan). These prostheses were used clinically from 1971 to 1978.

(2) Non-irradiated HDP socket with COP alloy head (28 mm)

(3) 100 Mrad irradiated HDP socket with an alumina head (28 mm)

The alumina head was attached by a taper on the stem made of COP alloy (Out of roundness < 1.0 μm, Surface roughness < 0.01 μm; Bioceram, Kyocera Co., Japan).

(4) UHMWPE socket with an alumina head (28mm)

Molecular weight of UHMWPE; 3,000,000–5,000,000.

(5) T-28. UHMWPE socket with a stainless-steel head (28 mm)

Molecular weight of UHMWPE ; 3,000,000–5,000,000.

The femoral components used were a mono block stem made of stainless steel (Out of roundness and surface roughness are unknown ; Zimmer Co.). Every femoral head size was 28 mm in diameter and every component was designed for cement fixation. We measured decreases in a thickness of the socket over 6 years. Cases for which the socket or stem loosened and the component shifted within 6 years, those not having well-defined radiographic reference points and those having metal-backed sockets were excluded from these measurements. Measurements were made of 28 COP alloy head (28 mm) with 100 Mrad irradiated HDP socket (COP-100 Mrad · HDP), 23 COP alloy head (28 mm) with 0 Mrad HDP socket (COP-0 Mrad · HDP), 12 Alumina head (28 mm) with 100 Mrad irradiated HDP socket (Alumina-100 Mrad · HDP), 111 Alumina head (28 mm) with 0 Mrad UHMWPE socket (Alumina-0 Mrad · UHMWPE), and T-28, stainless steel head (28 mm) with 2.5 Mrad UHMWPE socket (SUS-2.5 Mrad · UHMWPE) (Table 3).

2) Relationship between wear and thickness of the socket (28 mm alumina head with UHMWPE socket – total hip prosthesis)

In addition, we evaluated the relationship between wear and thickness of a UHMWPE socket articulating with an alumina ball (Bioceram, Kyocera Co.) in total hip prostheses, using measurements of wear on patient radiographs and on retrieved sockets. On measuring the radiographs, 111 joints in 102 cases were considered suitable for inclusion in this study; 14 joints in 13 cases were in males and 97 joints in 89 cases were in females. all cases were diagnosed as having secondary osteoarthritis due to a dysplastic acetabulum. 93 cases were unilateral and 9 cases were bilateral. Socket thickness ranged from 7 to 11 mm (Table 4).

With regard to the retrieved sockets, the prostheses were retrieved due to slight loosening of the stem, cup or both, or due to late infection between bone and components. Prostheses dam-

Table 3 Results of linear wear rate measurement in several kinds of prostheses measured on radiographs.

THP (28 mm Femoral Head)	Shape of Femoral Head	Linear Wear Rate (mm/year)	Number of Joints	Implanted Periods (years)
COP head with 100 Mrad irradiated HDP socket (COP-100 Mrad HDP)	O. R. > 10 μm S. R. > 0.5 μm	0.05 ± 0.04	28	6–23
COP head with 0 Mrad irradiated HDP socket (COP-0 Mrad HDP)	O. R. > 10 μm S. R. > 0.5 μm	0.29 ± 0.02	23	6–13
Alumina head with 100 Mrad irradiated HDP socket (Alumina-100 Mrad HDP)	O. R. < 1.0 μm S. R. < 0.01 μm	0.05 ± 0.03	12	14–16
Alumina head with 0 Mrad irradiated UHMWPE socket (Alumina-0 Mrad UHMWPE)	O. R. < 1.0 μm S. R. < 0.01 μm	0.10 ± 0.007	111	10–19
T28, stainless steel head with 2.5 Mrad UHMWPE socket (SUS-2.5 Mrad UHMWPE)	O. R. and S. R. Unknown	0.25 ± 0.02	15	6–15

HDP: Hoechst, molecular weight 1,000,000   COP: Stainless steel containing 20% cobalt
100 Mrad irradiated socket: Cross-linked socket irradiates with 100 Mrad gamma ray.
2.5 Mrad: Sterilized with 2.5 Mrad gamma ray.
O. R.: Out of roundness   S. R.: Surface roughness   * $P < 0.001$

Table 4 Results of relationship linear wear rate and thickness of the socket in total hip prosthesis of 28 mm-alumina head with UHMWPE socket measured on radiographs.

Socket thickness (mm)	Linear Wear Rate (mm/year)	Number of Joints
7	0.14 ± 0.10	22
8	0.15 ± 0.11	21
9	0.12 ± 0.03	21
10	0.06 ± 0.03	25
11	0.08 ± 0.04	22

aged by means other than wear by the femoral head were excluded from this study. Socket thickness and the number of retrieval cases, in which the inner surface could be measured, are shown in the Table 3.

Methods

1) Measurements of linear wear rate on radiographs

The linear wear was measured using a refinement of the method of Livermore (6) by means of a digi-

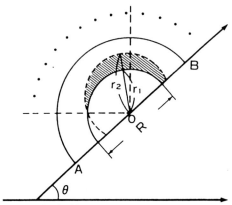

Fig. 6 Method of linear wears measurement
A, B: Outer edge of the socket. O: Center of socket.
R: Head diameter
R1: Head diameter measured at the index radiograph
R2: Head diameter measured in the follow up radiograph
r1, r2: Measured length from the socket center
Note that the measurement was done at 10 degree increment and the maximum value was used.
Linear wear = r2 x 28/R2 – r1 x 28/R1

tizer (20 μm resolution) and 5 × magnification viewing glass as previously reported. Briefly, the center of the socket was first identified as the mid-point of the long axis of the socket (shown by both ends of the circumferential marker wire in the sockets) and superior-medial displacement of the head center was defined as the linear wear (Figure 6). Measurements of displacement were performed at 10 degree intervals and the maximum value was used as the linear wear because this is the plane closest to the wear direction. Magnification was then corrected with reference to the head diameter. The wear rate was calculated as the value during the first two years (initial wear bedding-in), and thereafter (steady state wear), and statistically analyzed with analysis of variance (ANOVA) using a statistical software package (Stat View 4.5, Abacus Concepts Inc. Berkeley, California).

2) Measurements of linear wear rate on retrieved sockets

Generally, the inner surface of a retrieved socket has two spherical surfaces (Figure 7). Consequently, the distance between the center 0 of spherical surface I and the center 0' of spherical surface II was regarded to be the length of the

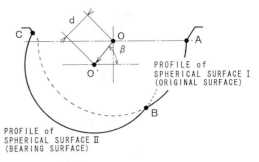

Fig. 8 Wear profile diagram
O: Center of spherical surface I.   O': Center of spherical surface II
d = Distance O – O' (linear wear)   β = Wear angle, measured from the plane of the mouth of the socket

femoral head movements during use, that is, wear including creep deformity of the polyethylene socket. This is called linear wear. The distance between 0 and 0' was defined as the length of the femoral head movement, d. The direction of movement was defined as the angle from the datum plane, β (Figure 8). In this case, the initial wear, which was much higher than the steady state wear, could not be excluded, thus, the wear rates recorded included the initial wear in the final steady state wear rate calculated.

Results

1) Comparisons of linear wear rate of several kinds of total hip prostheses

The linear wear rates are shown on the Table 3.
The linear wear rates of (1) COP-100 Mrad · HDP, (2) COP-0 Mrad · HDP, (3) alumina-100 Mrad · HDP, (4) alumina-0 Mrad · UHMWPE, and (5) SUS-2.5 Mrad · UHMWPE were 0.05 ± 0.04, 0.29 ± 0.02, 0.05 ± 0.03, 0.10 ± 0.007, and 0.25 ± 0.02 mm/year (mean ± SE), respectively.
The wear rate of COP-100 Mrad · HDP was significantly lower than that in COP-0 Mrad · HDP and SUS-2.5 Mrad · UHMWPE ($P < 0.0001$), and was half of that seen in alumina-0 Mrad · UHMWPE. The mean rates of COP-100 Mrad · HDP and alumina-100 Mrad · HDP were the same. The mean rate of alumina-0 Mrad · UHMWPE was less than half of SUS-2.5 Mrad · UHMWPE.

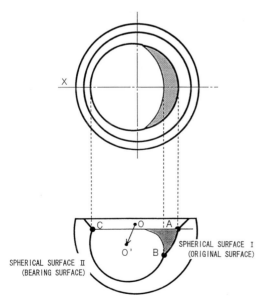

Fig. 7 Schematic drawing of the inner surface of the retrieved socket, showing the original surface and the bearing surface after wear.

2) Relationship between linear wear rate and thickness of the socket (28 mm alumina head with UHMWPE socket – total hip prosthesis)

a) The linear wear rate on radiographs

The average wear rates of the socket thickness of 7, 8, 9, 10, and 11 mm wear 0.14 ± 0.10, 0.15 ± 0.11, 0.12 ± 0.03, 0.06 ± 0.03, and 0.08 ± 0.04 mm/year, respectively (Table 4).

Scatter of the wear rates was very wide especially where the thickness of the socket was thin. The wear rates for the 7 and 8 mm thick sockets were almost the same and twice that of 10 and 11 mm thick sockets. The thicker the socket, the lower the wear rate ($P < 0.005$).

b) The linear wear rate of retrieved sockets

The linear wear rates of 7, 8, 9, and 11 mm thick sockets were 0.20 ± 0.03, 0.19 ± 0.01, 0.14 ± 0.08, and 0.10 ± 0.03 mm/year, respectively (Table 5). The wear rates of the 6 and 7 mm thick socket were almost the same and twice that of the 11 mm thick sockets. The thicker the socket, the lower the wear, as seen on the radiograph study ($P<0.005$).

Table 5 Results of relationship linear wear rate and thickness of the socket in total hip prosthesis of 28 mm-alumina head with UHMWPE socket measured on retrieved prostheses.

Socket thickness (mm)	Linear Wear Rate (mm/year)	Number of Joints
7	0.20 ± 0.03	4
8	0.19 ± 0.01	3
9	0.14 ± 0.08	5
11	0.10 ± 0.03	2

[II] Alumina Total Knee Prosthesis

In the clinical experience of total hip prostheses with 28-mm alumina heads against UHMWPE sockets since 1977, the decrease in the thickness of the socket against the alumina head was an average of 0.08 mm/year, while that against the metal heads was 0.3 mm/year.

Both experimental and clinical results indicated that the wear of the UHMWPE was significantly lower in the combination with alumina than with metal. These advantages led to the development of the alumina total knee prosthesis (KOM; KOKU-RITSU OSAKA-MINAMI HOSPITAL; author's hospital name). A combination of alumina and UHMWPE in the sliding portions was used.

The alumina ceramic total knee prosthesis, which uses alumina in the portions that come in contact with the bone at the beginning (the 1st generation) and uses a combination of alumina and UHMWPE in the portions that slide, is referred to as total condylar prosthesis. The stem is positioned at the center of the tibial plate, and the load is transmitted through the stem to the cortical bone in the posterior portion of the tibia (Figure 9 (a)).

Simulator Test

To know the mean resistance of alumina total knee prosthesis, a knee simulator was used. In the present study, wear tests were performed and comparisons were made between total knee prostheses that used alumina with UHMWPE and those that used Co-Cr-Mo alloy with UHMWPE, with and without metal trays. The three prostheses were similar in configuration. The maximum load was 20 MPa. The extent of anteroposterior (AP) movement of the femoral component on the tibial component was 5 mm. The flexion and extension angles of the knee were 15 and 0, respectively. One cycle of walking was 1.8 seconds. The number of repetitions was one million. The sliding portion was filled with a saline solution (Figure 10). The decrease in thickness was measured by contracer (Figure 11).

According to the simulator test results, the maximum decrease in thickness of the UHMWPE was 0.3 mm in the case of the combination with metal (total condylar), whereas no decrease in thickness was seen in many portions of the combination with alumina. The total decrease in thickness of UHMWPE in combination with alumina was less than one tenth that of the combination with metal (Figure 12).

Design

1) 1st generation (KOM-1) (January 1982–February 1985)

In the 1st generation, components were designed as a cementless. A tibial UHMWPE plate was fixed on the alumina tray. The stem of an alumina was positioned at the center of the tray, and the load was transmitted through the stem to the cortical bone in the posterior portion of the tibia. On the portion contacting the bone of both femoral and tibial components, small and shallow grooves were made. The both components of the

1.2 Concepts and Designs with Ceramics for Total Hip and Knee Replacement

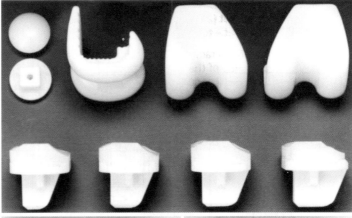

a The 1st generation

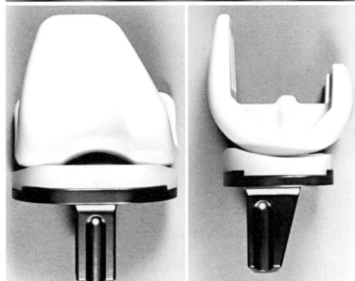

b The 2nd generation

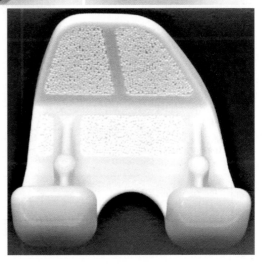

c The 3rd generation

Fig. 9a–c Alumina total knee prostheses

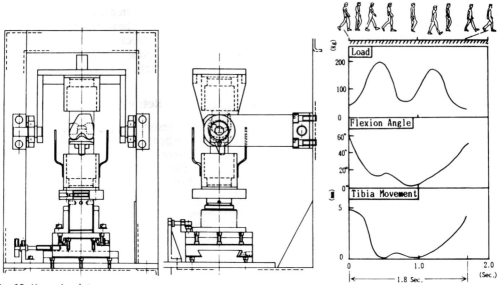

Fig. 10 Knee simulator

Fig. 11 Decrease in thickness of UHMWPE was measured by contracer

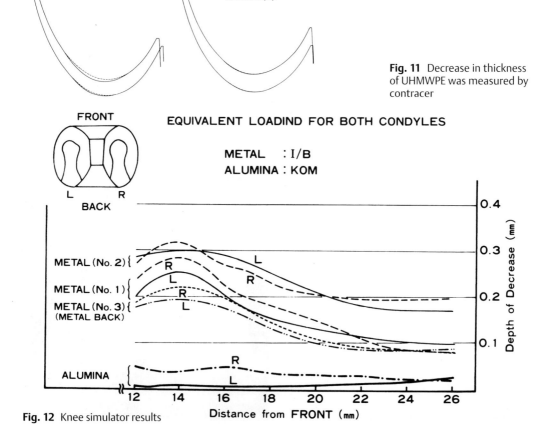

Fig. 12 Knee simulator results

femur and the tibia can be used as both a cementless and a cement fixation (Figure 9 (a)).

2) 2nd generation (KOM-2) (January, 1990–April, 1996)

In the 2nd generation, as an alumina tibial tray was thick and brittle, and the relatively high incidence of sinking and radiolucent lines in components without bone cement fixation was found in the 1st generation, an alumina tray was changed to titanium alloy tray which was fixed with bone cement (Figure 9 (b)).

3) 3rd generation (KOM-3) (March, 1993–October, 1998)

In the 3rd generation, a femoral component was coated with alumina beads to improve the cement fixation strength. Because the elastic modulus of an alumina and bone cement was extremely different (Figure 9 (c)).

Wear of the Retrieved Cases

When prosthesis loosens, its sliding part may become rough by three body wear, and a thick connective tissue membrane may be interposed between the component and bone. Therefore we observed three cases without loosening, includ-

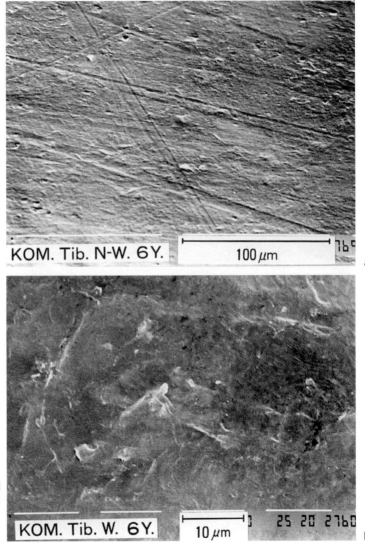

Fig. 13a,b Alumina Total Knee Prosthesis. SEM observed retrieved tibial UHMWPE plate. Postmortem case 6 years after surgery.
(a): Non-weight bearing area
(b): Weight bearing area

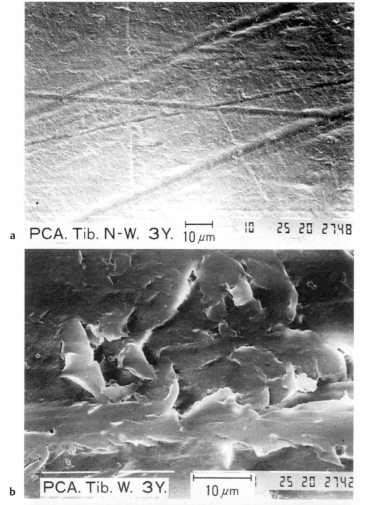

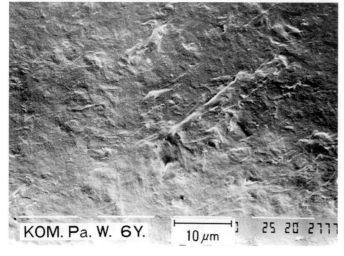

Fig. 14a,b Co-Cr-Mo (PCA) total knee prostheses. SEM observed retrieved tibial UHMWPE plate. Late infection case 3 years after surgery.
(a): Non-weight bearing area
(b): Weight bearing area

Fig. 15 SEM observed Retrieved patella UHMWPE on weight bearing area. Postmortem case 6 years after surgery.

1.2 Concepts and Designs with Ceramics for Total Hip and Knee Replacement

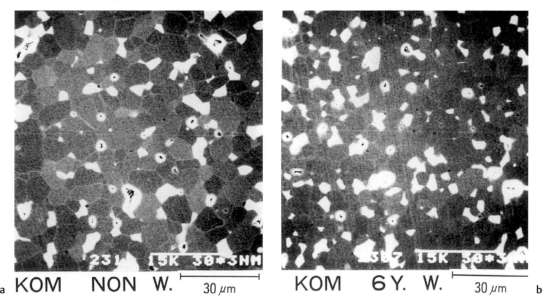

Fig. 16a,b Alumina total knee prosthesis. SEM observed retrieved alumina femoral condyle. Postmortem case 6 years after surgery. (a): Non-weight bearing area. (b): Weight bearing area

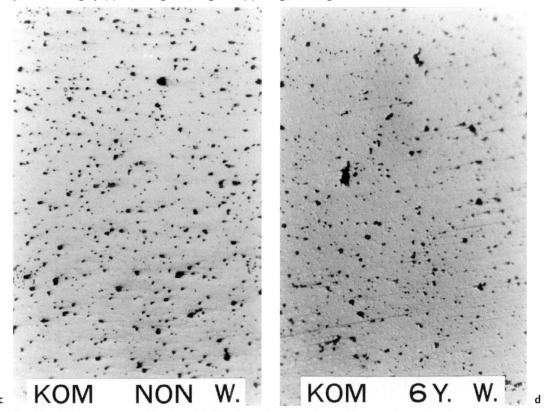

Fig. 16c,d The same case as Fig. 16 (a, b). Alumina surface was observed by metallographic microscope. (c): Non-weight bearing area. (d): Weight bearing area

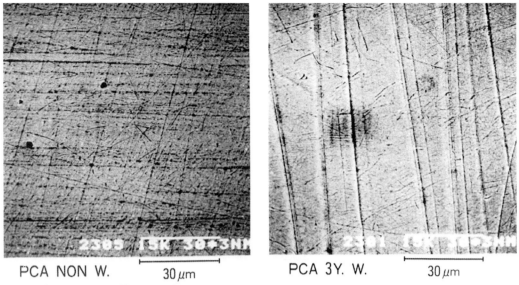

a PCA NON W. 30 μm PCA 3Y. W. 30 μm b

Fig. 17a,b Co-Cr-Mo total knee prosthesis. Retrieved Co-Cr-Mo femoral condyle was observed by SEM. Late infection case 3 years after surgery. (a): Non-weight bearing area. (b): Weight bearing area

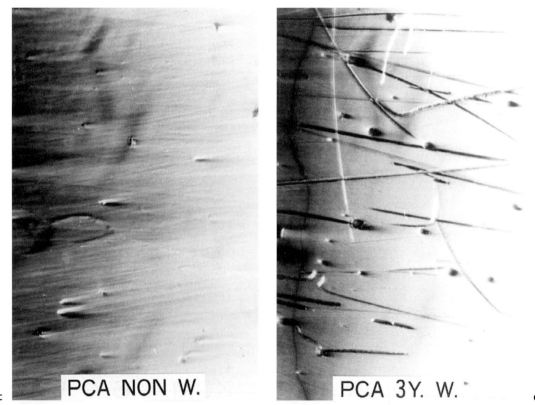

c PCA NON W. PCA 3Y. W. d

Fig. 17c,d The same case as Figure 17 (a, b). Co-Cr-Mo surface was observed by metallographic microscope. (c): Non-weight bearing area. (d): Weight bearing area

ing two cases postmortem (6 months and 6 years after implantation) and a case with infection between bone and component (1 year after implantation). We also observed another infected case of a non-loosening PCA made of a combination of Co-Cr-Mo alloy and UHMWPE (3 years after implantation). These patients all suffered rheumatoid arthritis, but could walk before removal. SEM observed the UHMWPE surfaces of tibial plates and patella components. SEM and a metallographic microscope observed the surfaces of femoral components. Histology observations of the surrounding tissues were performed by light microscopy.

1) UHMWPE surfaces of tibial plate

Alumina knee prosthesis were found to have gently sloping machine marks left, measuring one to several μm, on non-weight bearing areas, while machine marks on weight bearing areas completely disappeared 6 years after operation, though some remained in places at 6 months and 1 year after implantation. Overall observation revealed almost all surfaces were smooth and burnished without scratches or pits. The polyethylene folding phenomenon, which is thought to be caused by three-body wear occurring as a result of interposition of polyethylene wear particles between components, was also seen in places, though to a small extent. It was suspected that a part of the tip of this folded polyethylene was torn into debris when a force was transmitted onto the tip from the femoral component (Figure 13).

In the case of a PCA made of a combination of Co-Cr-Mo alloy and UHMWPE, burnishing was seen in sites where machine marks disappeared, and small scratches were observed at these sites 3 years after joint replacement. The folding phenomenon was observed frequently, and folding sites mingles with scratches in many places (Figure 14).

2) UHMWPE surfaces of patellar components

Since a tibial component has a concave or flat surface while a patellar component has a convex surface, the surface of the patellar component wears differently from that of a tibial component. Due to the convex shape, many artificial scratches were present over the surface; however, it was unclear when they occurred, before use, during implantation or at the time of removal. In sliding parts without artificial scratches, burnishing sites mingled with folding sites. It was especially noted that there were many dimples, measuring two to three μm in diameter. The Co-Cr-Mo alloy PCA case showed similar changes to those seen in the alumina knee prosthesis (Figure 15).

3) The surfaces of femoral components

In alumina femoral components, sliding parts in some areas appeared burnished by SEM observation, however no measurable change was observed by light microscopy (Figure 16). In contrast, observable burnishing and scratches were produced on sliding parts of the Co-Cr-Mo alloy PCA (Figure 17).

Fixation to the Bone

The 1st generation:

When the cementless fixation was performed, during surgery, the authors fill the space generated between the component and the bone with crushed bone, to make the connective tissue membrane that lies between the two structures as thin as possible and to prevent loosening. Specifically, place small pieces of bone on the metal tray that was developed on a trial basis, hammer the bone to prepare crushed bone, spread the crushed bone 2–3 mm in thickness over the surfaces of the bone just before installing the component, and then put the component in place.

The 2nd and 3rd generation:

To solve the interface problems of traditional PMMA bone cement, the author studied a method of making bioactive bone cement only at the interface by interposing 0 to two layers of fine and porous hydroxyapatite (HA) granules (100–300 μm diameter) between bone and PMMA cement

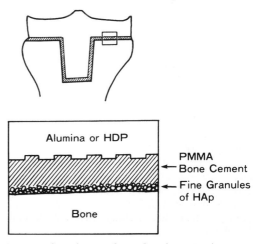

Fig. 18 The scheme of interface bioactive bone cement. (IBBC) technique

at surgery. The technique is called interface bioactive bone cementation (IBBC). When performed correctly, HA forms a strong union by physicochemically bonding with bone ingrowing into intervals between granules, and HA granules are mechanically linked to the bone cement. Hemostasis is very important while cementing 30–33, 39–42 (Figure 18).

The IBBC technique was performed in femoral condyles of rabbits. Over a period of 6 weeks following implantation, PMMA cement, HA granules, and bone were gradually replaced by their neighboring material or substance, not intermittently replaced (i.e., a functional gradient material at the interface). IBBC bonding strength between bone and material immediately after surgery was relatively strong, and at 6 and 12 weeks after surgery it was almost the same as that of materials with a HA coating on a smooth surface. Therefore, the IBBC technique is a bonding method that has advantages similar to those of both non-cemented fixation with HA coating and a traditional bone cement fixation.

Clinical Studies

1) The 1st generation

A marked bony atrophy, a marked sclerotic bone, and a large bone graft in the weight-bearing region were considered as contraindications for cements fixation. Components in tibias and femurs with marked bony atrophy will gradually sink after surgery. Therefore, fixation with bone cementless was performed. If the bone is markedly sclerotic and the space prepared by osteotomy or bone excision is slightly smaller than the component, fracture of the femoral component might occur on insertion because the bone cannot be deformed. Even if there is no problem on insertion, the contact area after insertion is extremely small and there are many spaces, resulting in poor fixation. One cannot expect new bone formation to occur in the spaces, even though they are filled with crushed bone, because bone fragments will often be absorbed under these circumstances. In these cases, cement fixation was performed. It is desirable to adjust the amount of excised bone when a large bone graft is required in the weight-bearing region. There is a high risk of destroying graft bone.

Alumina total knee arthroplasty was performed on 137 patients, including 103 with rheumatoid arthritis (RA) and 34 with osteoarthrosis of the knee (OA), from January 1982 to February 1985 (the 1st generation). In this clinical study, patients who could be evaluated by the end of December 1998 were used as subjects. During the follow-up period, 56 patients died (38 with RA and 18 with OA); 37 revisited the hospital for the follow-up roentgenographic examination (33 with RA and 4 with OA, including one RA patient with infection); 16 answered the questionnaire, but did not revisit for roentgenographic examination (13 with RA and 3 with OA); and 28 could not be evaluated (19 with RA and 9 with OA). One hundred eight patients did not have follow-up examinations; the follow-up rate was 80%.

The reasons why patients answered the questionnaire but did not revisit the hospital were as follows: some performed the activities of daily living without pain while walking, and some lived far from the hospital and had no one to help them come to the hospital. None of these patients reported difficulty in walking because of pain. Follow-up evaluations were not done because new addresses were not received after patients moved, or contact could not be made with patients who lived far from the hospital.

In this study, 37 patients with 61 involved knees (37 RA patients with 56 involved knees; 4 OA patients with 5 involved knees) who could have had a follow-up evaluation by the end of December 1998 were analyzed. From this study, one patient with infection (one with RA) was excluded. The RA patients ranged from 28 to 72 years of age, with a mean age of 54.6 years at the time of operation; the OA patients ranged from 54 to 74 years of age, with a mean age of 70 years. Follow-up periods at the end of December 1998 ranged from 13 years ten months to 16 years 11 months, with a mean of 15 years six months. In RA patients, the range was 13 years ten months to 16 years 11 months, with a mean of 15 years five months; in OA patients, the range was 14 years five months to 16 years eight months, with a mean of 15 years eight months.

Fixation with PMMA bone cement was performed on 10 of the 56 RA knees. None of the 5 OA knees were fixed with bone cement.

Result

In the group of the 1st generation, of the RA knees, 40 knees were roentgenographically measured, excluding 15 knees revised because of loosening

1.2 Concepts and Designs with Ceramics for Total Hip and Knee Replacement

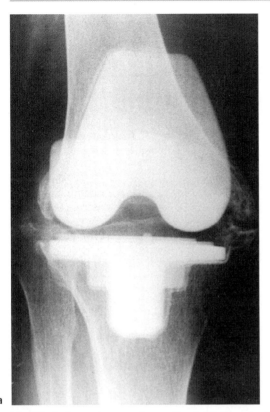 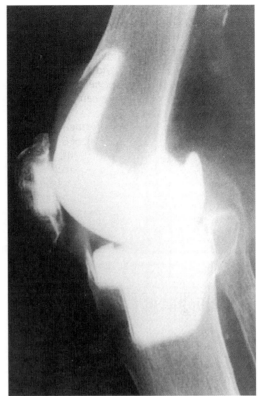

Fig. 19a,b Loosening case (cementless). RA. 71 year-old. Female. 9 years after surgery.

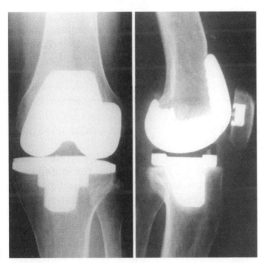 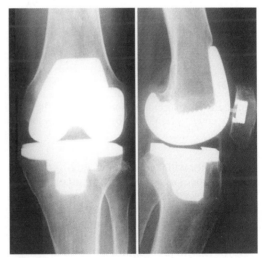

Fig. 20a,b No complication case (cementless). (a): one year after surgery. (b): 15 years after surgery.

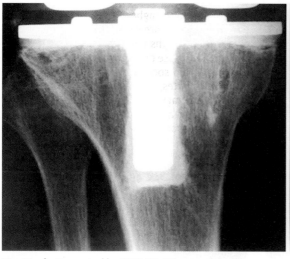 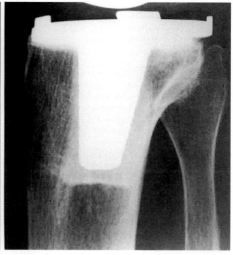

Fig. 21a,b Cemented by IBBC. RA. 10 years after surgery

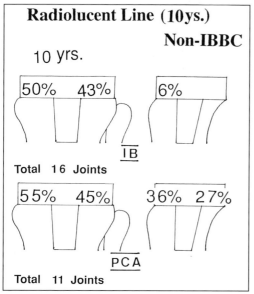 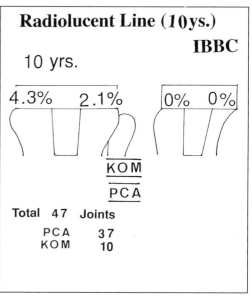

Fig. 22a,b Radiolucent line appearance rate 10 years after surgery
(a): Cemented by Non-IBBC. (b): Cemented by IBBC

and one knee with late infection. Among these 40 knees, 10 knees were fixed with bone cement, and 9 knees showed neither loosening nor sinking at all, although the remaining one exhibited loosening in both femoral and tibial components.

As for the 33 cases without bone cement fixation, the loosening or sinking, in the tibial component was found in 19 joints and no loosening or sinking was found in 12 joints. The loosening or sinking in the femoral component without bone cement fixation was found in 12 joints (Figure 19), and no loosening and sinking was found in 19 joints (Figure 20).

Of the OA knees, 3 knees were roentgenographically measured, excluding 2 knees revised because of loosening. As for the OA knees, loosening or sinking in the tibial components was found in 2 joints and no loosening or sinking was found in one joint. The loosening or sinking in femoral component was not found in 3 joints. In the groups of the 2nd and the 3rd generations, there was neither sinking nor loosening of the components. The radiolucent line appeared only on the small areas of few cases. There was no complication (Figure 21, 22).

Discussion

We compared the wear rate for several kinds of prostheses in this clinical study. The wear of a HDP socket articulating with crude a COP metal head was significantly reduced by 100 Mrad radiation of the HDP socket. 100 Mrad radiation of HDP has been proven to be effective in reducing wear rate not only experimentally but also clinically.

The wear rate of a non-cross-linked polyethylene socket articulating with an alumina head was 40% of that articulating with a metal heads. On the other hand, the wear rates of gamma irradiated cross-linked HDP sockets articulating with metal heads and with alumina heads were the same. In other words, the wear of the total hip prostheses was scarcely affected by material or quality of the femoral head, but was affected by the quality of the polyethylene socket.

As the cross-linked polyethylene socket used clinically was gamma-irradiate HDP in the air, the surface of the socket was oxidized and, as a result, the wear of the socket was affected. However, in our recent hip simulator tests using cross-linked UHMWPE sockets in which the surface oxidation was eliminated, articulating with an alumina ball, wear of the cross-linked socket was not defected after 6 million cycles.

Concerning the relationship between wear rate and socket thickness with 28 mm alumina head in our clinical cases, the wear rates of 7 mm and 8 mm thick sockets were almost the same and twice of that of the 10 and 11 mm thick socket. The thicker the polyethylene socket, the lower the wear rates. In this study the number of the cases was not enough to make a final conclusion. Scatter of wear rate was very wide, especially, in the case of radiographs, where the thickness of the socket was thinner. In the case of radiographs, the wear rate of 8 mm sockets was somewhat higher than that of 7 mm. In addition, the wear rate of 11 mm sockets was higher than that of 10 mm sockets. If we had more cases, the average wear rate line on the graphs might have become a sloping curve. If one case of a 8 mm socket and two cases of the 11 mm sockets, which showed extremely high wear rates, are excluded from the population, the average line on the graph will be nearer to sloping or a straight line. In our previous reports, it was found that the thicker the polyethylene socket, the lower the wear rates. When a socket of 9 mm in thickness was used, the linear wear rates of the polyethylene socket articulating on the 22, 28 and 32 mm femoral heads were almost the same. When a socket over 11 mm in thickness was used, the volumetric wear rates were almost the same.

The decrease in thickness of UHMWPE (a sum of wearing and creeping deformation) in tibial plate was compared with the total condylar knee prosthesis made of a combination of Co-Cr-Mo alloy and UHMWPE and the KOM made of a combination of alumina and UHMWPE in a knee simulator test. This revealed that the amount of decrease in UHMWPE thickness in combination with alumina was as small as one tenth of that seen in combination with Co-Cr-Mo alloy.

When the retrieved tibial plates were compared with respect to changes in UHMWPE caused by friction and wearing between a combination with alumina and that with Co-Cr-Mo alloy, it was noted that not only did the wearing patterns differ, but also the surface of the latter combination showed more remarkable changes. Changes in UHMWPE surfaces examined in the simulator test agreed with those seen clinically. Furthermore, when weight-bearing surfaces of femoral components were observed under SEM, the alumina surface showed very slight changes while the Co-Cr-Mo alloy surface had scratches.

Based on these results, it was assumed that the decrease in thickness of UHMWPE on a tibial plate was smaller in a combination with alumina than with Co-Cr-Mo alloy, although the amount of decrease in thickness could not be roentgenographically measured. It should be noted that the decrease in thickness of a UHMWPE socket of a total hip prosthesis was previously measured using roentgenographs and found that the amount in combination with an alumina head was about one third that with a metal head.

When the surfaces of UHMWPE in pateller components in combination with alumina and with Co-Cr-Mo alloy were compared, the folding phenomenon was frequently seen in both combinations, showing no differences. This indicated that patellar components wore rapidly because of the convex shape.

In the 1st generation, in clinical cases, neither clear zones nor sinking appeared when the components were fixed with bone cement, except in one case. This case had RA of the mutilans-type, known to frequently cause sinking and loosening. The reasons for the relatively high incidence of sinking and clear zones in components without bone-cement fixation were thought to be that tibial component was often smaller than tibial surface in early days. Because a sufficient number of sizes was not available at that time, and that most of the cases had RA, which was classified as the mutilans-type. Therefore, it is desirable to perform bone-cement fixation in these situations. It has frequently been reported that alumina has excellent biocompatibility and bonding with bone. This has been conformed by animal experiments. However, follow-up roentgenographic examinations have disclosed that alumina is not always superior to metal or polymeric materials in bonding with bone. Alumina is completely inert and extremely stable in the body. However, a complicated and fine design with alumina cannot be realized. To firmly fix alumina to the bone, as with other materials, the anchorage of the prosthesis requires excellent mechanical fixation such as that achieved with screws or through porous surfaces. At present, the reason for using alumina is the excellent wear resistance of the UHMWPE against this ceramic in the sliding part. This is more important than alumina being inert in vivo.

In the 2nd and the 3rd generations, for fixation to the bone IBBC technique (Interface Bioactive Bone Cement) was used. By this technique bone and bone cement was bound physico-chemically after bone in growth into the HA particles interposed between bone and bone cement, and HA particles and bone cement was bound immediately after cementation. In consequent, bone and bone cement was bound physicochemically by interposing HA particles.

IBBC technique had been used over 2,000 cases in total hip and knee arthroplasty since 1987. Radiolucent line appeared on the small area in the few cases. There was no loosening. IBBC has the both advantages of bone cement fixation and HA coating cementless fixation, and could be expected to have long term fixation.

In the 3rd generation, stronger fixation between alumina and bone cement can be obtained as the beads were coated on the alumina. In our recent hip stimulator studies, we have found the wear of alumina on alumina total hip prostheses to be extremely low (0.004 $mm^3/10^6$ cycles). Consequently, for a while, we will use both an alumina on alumina total hip prosthesis and an alumina on an irradiated cross-linked UHMWPE total hip prosthesis. In the future, we hope to find which is better from these clinical results and to find optimum doses of irradiation on UHMWPE in combination with alumina or zirconia total knee prosthesis.

Reference

1 *Chmell, M.J., Poss, R., Thomas, W.H., Sledge, C.B.*: Early failure of Hylamer acetabular inserts due to eccentric wear. J. Arthroplasty 11: (1996) 351–353
2 *Clarke, I.C., Good, V., Williams, P., Oparaango, P., Oonishi, H. et al.*: Simulator wear study of High dose gamma-irradiated UHWMPE cups. Trans. Soc. Biomater. 20: (1997) 71
3 *Clarke, I.C.*: Ceramic on ceramic total hip prosthesis. the 28th Annual Meeting of the Japanese Society for Replacement Arthroplasty, March 5–6 (1998), Kanazawa/Japan
4 *Holowitz, S.M., Doty, S.B., Lane, J.M., Burstain, A.H.*: Studies of the mechanism by which the mechanical failure of polymethylmethacrylate leads to bone resorption. J. Bone Joint Surg. (Am) 75-A: (1993) 802–813
5 *Kadoya, Y., Revell, P.A., Al-Saffar, N., Kobayashi, A., Scott, G. et al.*: Wear particulate species and bone loss in failed total joint arthroplasties. Clin. Orthop. 340: (1997) 118–129
6 *Levermore, J., Ilstrup, D., Morrey, B.*: Effect of femoral head size on wear of the polyethylene acetabular component. J. Bone Joint Surg. (Am) 72A: (1990) 518–528
7 *Livingston, B.J., Chmell, M.J., Spector, M., Poss, R.*: Complications of total hip srthroplasty associated with the use of an acetabular component with a Hylamer Liner. J. Bone Joint Surg. (Am) 79-A: (1997) 1529–1538
8 *Okumura, H., Yamamuro, T., Kawai, T., Nakamura, T.*: Socket wears in total hip prostheses with alumina ceramic head. Bioceramics 1: (1989) 284–289
9 *Oonishi, H., Hasegawa, T.*: Cementless alumina ceramic total knee prosthesis. Orthopedic Ceramic Implants 1: (1981) 157–160
10 *Oonishi, H., Kawaguchi, A., Tatsumi, M.*: Biomechanical analysis of the knee replaced with cementless alumina ceramic artificial knee joint – by means of 3D-FEM. Orthopedic Ceramic Implants 2: (1982) 61–84
11 *Oonishi, M., Kawaguchi, A., Tatsumi, M.*:Biomechanical analysis of the knee replaced with cementless

alumina ceramic artificial knee joint by means of 3D-FEM. Orthop. Ceram. Implants 2: (1982) 61
12. *Oonishi, H., Shikita, T.*: Alumina ceramic total hip prosthesis. Bessatsu Seikei-Geka No.3: (1983) 264–279, Nankodo (Japanese)
13. *Oonishi, H., Tatsumi, M.*: Some biomechanical considerations of finite element analysis of cementless alumina ceramic total knee prosthesis. In Biomaterial and Biomechanics, Amsteerdam, Elsevier, (1983) 49–54
14. *Oonishi, H., Maeda, A., Murata, N., Nabeshima, T.*: Designs and surgical technique of ouor cementless alumina ceramic total knee prosthesis. Jap. J. Rheum. Joint Surg. II:(1) (1983) 11–18
15. *Oonishi, H., Tatsumi, M.*: Some biomechanical considerations of finite element analysis of cementless alumina ceramic total knee prostheses. Biomaterials and Biomechanics (1983), Elsevier, Amsterdam, (1984) 49–54
16. *Oonishi, H., Okabe, N., Nabeshima, T., Kushitani, S., Tsuyama, K.*: Some problems of cementless alumina ceramic total knee prosthesis and its solutions. Orthopaedic Ceramic Implants 4: (1984) 275–288
17. *Oonishi, H., Nabeshima, T., Hanatate, Y., Tsuji, E.*: Wear test of KOM-alumina total knee prosthesis by a knee simulator. Orthopoaedic Ceramic Implants 4: (1984) 297–304
18. *Oonishi, H., Maeda, A., Hamaguchi. T., Nabeshima, T.*: Indications for cementless alumina ceramic total knee prosthesis and its limitation. Jap. Rheum. Joint Surg. III, 4: (1984) 311–322
19. *Oonishi, H. et al.*: Finite element analysis of an uncemented alumina ceramic total kneeprosthesis. Biomaterials '84 Transactions, Vol. VII (1984) 118
20. *Oonishi, H.*: Biomechnaical analysis of cementless alulmina ceramic total knee prosthesis with reference to clinical experience. Research MA J VI 2: (1985) 1–18
21. *Oonishi, H. et al.*: Comparison of wear test of KOM alumint-to UHMWPE and metal-to-UHMWPE total knee prosthesis by a knee simulator. Transactions of the 5th European Conference on Biomaterials, (1985) 79
22. *Oonishi, H., Maeda, A., Murata, N., Kushitani, S., Aono, M., Nabeshima, T., Tsuyama, K., Takayama, Y.*: An uncemented alulmina ceramic total knee prosthesis. In: Niewa S, Paul JP, Yamamoto S (eds) Total Knee Replacment. Springer, Berlin Heidelberg New York Tokyo, (1987) 193–205
23. *Oonishi, H. et al.*: Comparison of wear of slumina-to-UHMWPE and metal-to-UHMWPE total knee prosthesis by a knee simulator. Transactions of the second Japan-U.S.A.-China Conference on Biomechanics, (1987) 52
24. *Oonishi, H., Igaki, H., Takayama, Y.*: Comparison of wear of UHMWPE sliding against metal and alumina in total hip prostheses – Wear test and clinical results. Third World Biomaterials Congress, Transactions 337, April 21–25 (1988), Kyoto/Japan
25. *Oonishi, H. et al.*: An uncemented alumina ceramic total knee prosthesis. Total Knee Replacement, Springer-Verlag, (1988) 193–205
26. *Oonishi, H. et al.*: Interface bioactive bone cement by using PMMA and hydroxyapatite granules. Bioceramics Vol. 1, edited by Oonishi H, et al. Kyoto Japan, Ishiyaku Euro-America, Inc., Tokyo-St. Louis, (1989) 102–107
27. *Oonishi, H. et al.*: Comparisons of wear of UHMW polyethylene sliding against metal and alumina in total knee prostheses. Bioceramics Vol. 1, edited by Oonishi H, et al. Kyoto Japan, Ishiyaku Euro-America, Inc., Tokyo-St. Louis, (1989) 219–224
28. *Oonishi, H. et al.*: Interfacae bioactive bone cement technique of interposing hydroxyapatite granules between bone and PMMA bone cement –Experimental and clinical results –. Medical Engineering UK/Japan Biomaterials Symposium (1989)
29. *Oonishi, H., Igaki, H., Takayama, Y.*: Wear resistance of gamma-ray irradiated UHMW polyethylene socket in total hip prosthesis – Wear test and long term clinical results. MRS International Meeting on Advanced Materials, 1: (1989) 351–356
30. *Oonishi, H., Kushitani, S., Aono, M., Maeda, E., Tsuji, E., Ishimaru, H.*: Interface bioactive bone cement by using PMMA and hydroxyapatite granules. In: Bioceramics, Vol. 1, Ishiyaku-Euro-America, (1989) 102–107
31. *Oonishi, H. et al.*: Experimental and clinical results of interface bioactive bone cement. Bioceramics, 2: (1990) 410–417 (German Ceramic Society)
32. *Oonishi, H.*: Mechanical and chemical bonding of artificial joints. Interfaces in Biomaterials Sceinces, Proceedings of Symposium on Interface in Biomaterials Sciences of the 1989, E-MRS Conference, (1990) 121–137
33. *Oonishi, H., Kushitani, S., Ishimaru, H., Tsuji, E., Aono, M.*: A technique for interface bioactive bone cementation by interposing hydroxyapatite. In: Handbook of bioactive ceramics, Vol. 2, CRC, Boca Raton, (1990) 355–362
34. *Oonishi, H.*: Knee and ankle joint replacement. In: Osseo-Integrated Implants, vol. 1, CRC, Boca Raton, (1990) 171–186
35. *Oonishi, H., Tsuji, E., Hanatate, Y., Mizukoshi, T.*: Tribological studies on retrieved total joint prostheses outlines. Jpn. J. Tribol. 36(12): (1991) 1345–1355
36. *Oonishi, H.*: Orthopaedic ceramic implant; Japan clinical exsperiences. In: Material Science Monographs '69, Ceramics in Substitute and Reconstructive Surgery, Elsevier, Amsterdam, (1991) 623–638
37. *Oonishi, H., Tsuji, E., Mizukoshi, T., Fujisawa, A., Murata, N., Kushitani, S., Aono, M., Meguro, Y.*: Wear of polyethylene and alulmina in clinical cases of alumina total knee prostheses. In: Boceramics, Vol. 3, (1991) 137–145
38. *Oonishi, H., Aono, M.*: Clinical results of total knee arthroplasty in combination with alumina against polyethylene – a five to eight year follow up study. In: Boceramics, Vol. 3, (1991) 147–156
39. *Oonishi, H.*: Mechanical and chemical bonding of artificial joints. Clinical Materials, 5: (1991) 217–233
40. *Oonishi, H.*: Interfacial reactions to bioactive and non-bioactive bone cements. In: The bone biomate-

rial interface. University of Toronto Press, (1991) 321–333
41 *Oonishi, H.*: Bioceramics in orthopaedic surgery – Our clinical experiences. Bioceramics, 3, (1991) 31–42
42 *Oonishi, H.*: Interface bioactive bone cement as functional gradient materials. Bioceramics, 3: (1991) 243–253
43 *Oonishi, H.*: Wear of polyethylene and alumina in clinical cases of alumina total knee prostheses. Bioceramics, 3: (1991) 137–145
44 *Oonishi, H.*: Clinical results of total knee arthroplasty in combination with alumina against polyethylene – A five to eight year follow-up study. Boceramics, 3: (1991) 147–156
45 *Oonishi, H.*: Tribological studies on retrieved total joint prostheses outlines. Japanese Journal of Tribology, 36(12): (1991) 1345–1355
46 *Oonishi, H., Tsuji, E.*: In-vivo and in-vitro wear behaviour of alumina ceramics and UHMWPE implant bearing surface in total joint prostheses. In: Surface Modification technology, V. The Institute of Materials, (1992) 61–76
47 *Oonishi, H., Takayama, Y., Tsuji, E.*: In-vivo and in-vitro behaviour on weightbearing surface of polyethylene socket improved by irradiation in total hip prostheses. In: Surface Modification Technology, V. The Institute of Materials (1992) 101–115
48 *Oonishi, H., Takayama, Y., Tsuji, E.*: Improvement of polyethylene by irradiation in artificial joints, Rediation Physics and Chemistry 39(6): (1992) 495–504
49. *Oonishi, H., Takayama, Y., Clark, I.C., Jung, H.*: Comparative wear studies of 28-mm ceramic and stainless steel total hip joints over 2 to 7 year period. Journal of Long-Term Effects of Medical Implants 2(1): (1992) 37–47
50 *Oonishi, H., Takayama, Y., Tsuji, E.*: Improvement of polyethylene by irradiation in artificial joints. Radiat. Phys. Chem., 39(6): (1992) 495–504
51 *Oonishi, H., Takayama, Y.*: Comparative wear studies of 28-mm ceramic and steel total hip joints over 2 to 7 years. J. Long-Term Eff. Med. 2: (1992) 37–47
52 *Oonishi, H., Aono, M., Murata, N., Kushitani, S.* : Alumina versus polyethylene in total knee arthroplasty. Clinical Orthop. and Related Research, 282: (1992) 95–104
53 *Oonishi, H., Takayama, Y.*: In vivo and in vitro wear behabiour of alumina ceramic and UHMWPE implant bearing surfaces in total joint prostheses. Surface Modification Technologies V. Proceedings of the 5th International Conference, Edited by Sudarshan TS, The Institute of Materials, (1992) 61–76
54 *Oonishi, H., Aono, M., Murata, N., Kushitani, S.*: Alumina veersus polyethylene in total knee arthroplasty. Clinical Orthopaedics and Related Research, 282: (1992) 95–104
55 *Oonishi, H.*: Long term results of alumina total knee replacement. J. of Joint Surgery, 15(2): (1996) 41–52 (Japanese)
56 *Oonishi, H.*: New topics in TKA, a new concept on enduring total knee arthroplasty-low wear and adequate fixability to bone. Recostruction of the knee joint, edited by Niwa S, Yoshino S, et al., Springer-Verlag, (1997) 300–808
57 *Oonishi, H., Tsuji, E., Kim, Y.Y.*: Retrieved total hip prostheses, Part 1, The effects of cup thickness, head sizes and fusion defects on wear. J.of Materials Science ; Materials in Medicine, 9: (1998) 393–401
58 *Oonishi, H., Iwaki, H.K., Kin, N., Kushitani, H., Murata, N., Wakitani, S., Imoto, K.*: The effects of polyethylene cup thickness on wear of total hip prostheses. J. of Materials Science ; Materials in Medicine, 9: (1998) 475–478
59 *Ries, M.D., Bellare, A., Livingston, B.J., Cohen, R.E., Spector, M.*: Early delamination of a Hylamer-M tibial insert. J. Arthroplasty 11 : (1996) 974–976
60 *Schmalzried, T.P., Kwong, L.M., Jasty, M., Sedlacek, R.C., Haire, T.C. et al.*: The mechanism of loosening of cemented acetabular components in total hip arthroplasty ; analysis of specimens retrieved at autopsy. Clin. Orthop. 274: (1992) 60–78
61 *Schmalzried, T.P, Jasty, M., Harris, W.H.*: Periprosthetic bone loss in total joint hip arthroplasty ; the role of polyethylene wear debris and the concept of effective joint space. J. Bone Joint Surg. (Am) 74-A: (1992) 849–863
62 *Willert, H.G., Ludwig, J., Semlitsch, M.*: Reaction of bone to methacrylate after hip arthroplasty. A long-term gross, lightmicroscopic, and scanning electron microscopic study. J. Bone Joint Surg. (Am) 56-A: (1974) 1368–1382

1.3 The Transcend Alumina Ceramic Hip Articulation System
Surgical Technique – Preliminary Results of 51 cases

Marc Goossens

Introduction

In modern hip arthroplasty, fixation of the components – cemented or cementless – no longer appears to be the major issue of concern. Polyethylene wear is the common enemy. Polyethylene wear is a three-dimensional process that generates debris. Although all data regarding wear should be considered as estimates, it is agreed that the average linear wear of polyethylene liners varies between 0,1 and 0,2 mm per year (1). The important point is that polyethylene wear particles may induce a tissue reaction and osteolysis at the bone-implant interface and beyond, provoking loosening of the components and large bone defects. Assessment of wear is possible through a series of measurements. Linear wear can be measured on radiographs or via simulator tests, volumetric wear on retrieved components or through calculations from linear wear. With respect to linear wear, the polyethylene / metal combination appears to be the most unsuitable, with a mean wear rate of 200 microns a year (1,2). Modern metal-on-metal and ceramic-on-ceramic bearings perform much better (2,3) with wear rates as low as one micron per year for the Biolox forte combination (fig.1).

Ceramic bearings are not new and have been used for over 25 years. The early non-cemented ceramic cups were monolithic types like the Mittelmeier and Lindenhof. Although excellent results were reported by some designers, it became clear that the failure rate of these implants was high (4).

The problems are now well defined:

1. wear of the ceramic components, often due to vertical cup inclination,
2. fracture of ceramic balls, due to poor quality or taper mismatch and
3. migration and loosening, due to poor initial fixation.

Over the years, there has been a considerable improvement in the production of ceramics with regard to sphericity, surface polishing and taper technology. More recently, the Ceralock concept (1986) and the Biolox forte wear couple were introduced, resulting in modular ceramic-on-ceramic hip replacement systems (5).

The purpose of this study is to report the early experience with the ceramic-on-ceramic Transcend system (Wright Medical Technology, Arlington,TN, USA).

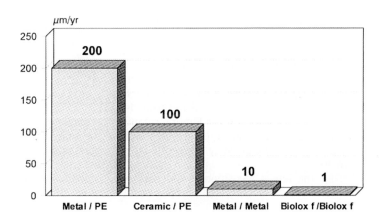

Fig. 1 Annual linear wear (after 1,2,3)

Material and Methods

The Transcend cup is a two-piece metal/ceramic cup. The titanium metal shell is designed as a press-fit cup with a porous coating for bone apposition. According to the Ceralock concept, the ceramic liner locks into the cup via a morse type taper. Femoral ceramic heads are available in 28, 32 and 36 mm. These come in three lengths resulting in a head size range of 7 mm.

Surgical technique

The surgical technique is similar to implanting a conventional system. However, one has to be aware of some pitfalls. Preoperative templating is essential for the obvious reason that there is only a 7 mm range in head size.

A direct lateral Hardinge approach is used on a patient in a supine position. According to the templating, a conservative neck cut is performed. The acetabulum should be exposed 360°. Acetabular reaming is started medially in order to restore the normal anatomy and to medialize the acetabular component. Subchondral bone support should be preserved at all times, as well as the acetabular walls.

The acetabular metal shell is positioned in 45° or less abduction and in 5 to 10° anteversion. Excessive vertical orientation of the shell should be avoided as this may lead to premature wear of the ceramics. At this point, an insert trial can be placed into the shell for trial reduction. Osteophytes are removed if necessary. The shell is cleared of any blood, soft tissue or bone debris. The ceramic insert is implanted in the shell by hand or by using the positioner-impactor device. While assembling the insert into the shell, tilting must be avoided at all times. As ceramic is a brittle material, excessive forces should never be used. A correctly placed insert will seat completely using minimal or no force at all. Seating can be checked by using the finger for palpation.

On the femoral side, a cemented stem without a collar is implanted. The absence of a collar offers a last resource for minor corrections regarding instability or leg length. A 28 mm femoral ceramic head is placed onto the stem by hand with a slight pressure and twist, followed by one gentle tap of the mallet.

Finally, the hip is repositioned and checked again for stability, mobility and absence of impingement.

Patient demographics

Between October 15, 1997 and December 18, 1998, 51 ceramic Transcends were implanted in 49 patients. There were two bilateral cases. A Perfecta plasma spray stem (Wright Medical Technology, Arlington, TN, USA) was cemented in 50 total hips, in one case a non-cemented cone prosthesis (Sulzer, Switzerland) was used.

The study is conducted as a prospective, non-randomized series. Indications for a ceramic-on-ceramic hip replacement include: patients younger than 60 years old, active patients under 70 years of age, small acetabula to avoid a thin PE liner, and on patients' request.

The demographic characteristics of the studied population are listed in Table 1. The mean age is 53 years old and the most common diagnosis is osteoarthritis (80%). Avascular necrosis was noted in seven hips (14%) in five patients (two bilateral cases).

Table 1 Demographics: Total number of patients = 51.

Male/Female	26/23
Right/Left	22/29
Means Age (yrs)	53 (27–73)
Mean Weight (kg)	77 (48–103)
Mean Length (cm)	170 (156–182)

Results

Clinical results are evaluated using the Harris Hip Score (HHS). As listed in Table 2, the HHS shows a pattern of gradual improvement, as in conventional hip systems, with a mean score of 98 points at one year post-operatively.

Table 2 Clinical Results – Harris Hip Scores.

Evaluation	Nr of Patients	Pain	Function	Overall HHs
preop	51	17	29	46
2 mos	51	41	43	84
6 mos	32	41	51	92
1 year	10	42	56	98

Radiographically, no adverse reactions are seen. No radiolucent lines were noted at the socket-bone interface. Cup migration or inclination was not observed at one year follow-up.

Shell positioning is crucial. An abduction angle of 45° is optimal. Fig. 2 shows the distribution of the abduction angle. The mean inclination angle

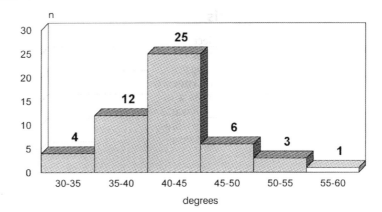

Fig. 2 Distribution of the cup inclination angle (mean = 42,8°)

was 42,8°. At least one cup was placed too vertically (56°). This cup might be at risk as the vertical position may load the edge of the insert, increasing the wear.

To evaluate leg lengthening, the distance between the acetabular roof and the lesser trochanter was measured pre- and post-operatively and compared with the opposite, healthy leg. The mean values of these measurements indicate that the leg shortening was overcorrected. As compared to the opposite side, the leg was lengthened by a mean of 6,8 mm.

Complications

The short-term complications encountered were two non-fatal lung embolisms despite prevention with Enoxaparin, three dislocations and one split-off of the rim of the ceramic inlay.

The dislocation pattern was similar in all 3 cases. They occurred after discharge from the hospital, three to four weeks post-op, with the patient doing an exorotation-adduction movement. Closed repositioning was performed without any additional bracing. None of the dislocations reoccurred. As the first and the third hip of the Transcend series dislocated, the dislocation rate must be considered as part of a learning curve. Since then, the anteversion angle of the cup was limited to 5 to 10°. Larger head diameters are also available for increased stability. However, in this series, only 28 mm heads were used for study purposes.

There was one splinter-fracture of the rim of the ceramic inlay. This complication must be considered as a technical failure and not as an implant failure. The liner was slightly tilted during insertion into the metal shell. Trying to correct this with a gentle mallet tap resulted in correct positioning, but also in a crack and a local fracture at the rim of the insert.

Discussion

The very low wear rates of the alumina ceramic couple are very promising. However, late complications as cup migration or wear and osteolysis may occur, even with ceramic bearings.

In a recent publication, cups with ceramic inlays were compared to cups with polyethylene inlays (6). Migration was significantly higher for the cups with the ceramic inlays. Progressive socket inclination occurred in four cups with ceramic inlays versus one cup with a polyethylene inlay. The authors conclude that the stiffness of ceramic liners influences the migration behaviour.

Another publication warns for the possibility of osteolysis with ceramic surfaces (7). Ceramic wear particles seem to stimulate a foreign body response and periprosthetic osteolysis. However, these findings were associated with the older Mittelmeier design.

Conclusions

Preliminary results with a new ceramic-on-ceramic system are encouraging.

Surgical technique is critical.

One should be aware of possible adverse reactions on the long term.

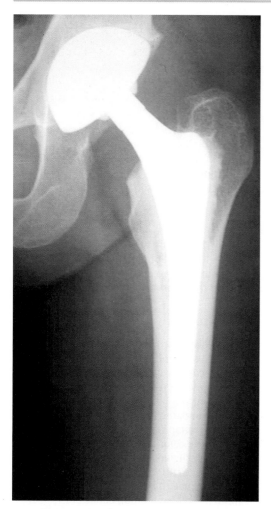

Fig. 3 The X-ray at one year shows the ceramic-on-ceramic hip articulation with a Transcend cup and a cemented stem.

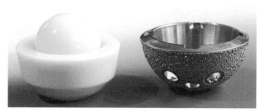

Fig. 4 The Transcend ceramic-on-ceramic cup design with the titanium shell, the ceramic insert and the ceramic ball head.

References

1. Zichner LP, Willert H-G: Comparison of Alumina-Polyethylene and Metal-Polyethylene in Clinical Trials. Clinical Orthopaedics and Related Research, 282, 86–94, 1992.
2. Streichner RM, Semlitsch M, Schön R, Weber BG, Rieker G: Metal-on-Metal Articulations for Artificial Hip Joints: Laboratory Study and Clinical Results. Proc. Instn. Mech. Engrs 210, 223, 1996.
3. Walter A: Investigation of the Wear Couple BIOLOX forte / BIOLOX forte. In: Puhl W (ed): Performance of the Wear Couple BIOLOX forte in Hip Arthroplasty. Enke Verlag. Stuttgart, 1997.
4. Clarke IC: Role of Ceramic Implants. Design and Clinical Success with Total Hip Prosthetic Ceramic-to-Ceramic Bearings. Clinical Orthopaedics and Related Research, 282, 19–30, 1992.
5. Willmann G.: Ceramics for Total Hip Replacement – What a Surgeon Should Know. Orthopedics, Vol 21, No 2, 173–177, 1998.
6. Boehler M, Mühlbauer M, Krismer M, Salzer M, Mayr G: Migration Measurements of Cementless Acetabular Components: Value of Clinical and Radiographic Data. Orthopedics, Vol 21(8), 897–900, 1998.
7. Yoon TR, Rowe SM, Jung ST, Seon KJ, Maloney WJ.: Osteolysis in Association with a Total Hip Arthroplasty with Ceramic Bearing Surfaces. Journal of Bone and Joint Surgery, Vol 80-A, No 10, 1459–1467, 1998.

1.4 Long-term Experience with the GSP and Anca Fit System

R. Alessandrini, G. Ghidoni, E. Tinelli, G. Giaretta

From October 1993 up to 31st December 1998 our department performed 1097 hip implants.

Out of these 49% (535) concerned hybrid prostheses, 44% (483) uncemented prostheses and 7% (79) revision prostheses.

For uncemented arthroprostheses we used GSP stems assembled with ANCA monobloc threaded ceramic cups with titanium threaded ring until the beginning of 1996, when we switched to the press-fit cup (Anca-fit) with inlay in Al_2O_3 and Anca fit stem derived from the GSP stem.

As for the revision prostheses we used the prostheses called Profemur.

Both GSP and Anca fit prostheses use the Biolox forte ceramic-ceramic coupling.

For the Profemur we used both press-fit cups with ceramic inlays and, in case of serious bone reabsorption, cups fixed by means of screws and with polyethylene inlays.

The prosthesis we use in our department has the advantage of being composed of a stem and a cup as close as possible to the anatomic reality of each patient.

To meet with this exigency we use modular prostheses.

The first expression of modularity in prosthetic stems was the introduction of modular heads with the possibility of using three different lengths of neck.

Afterwards Cremascoli enhanced its range of products (for both first implants and revisions) by adding to it necks of various lengths and angles.

This thanks to the introduction of the neck-stem assembly by means of an elliptical morse cone, which grants a stronger resistance to the rotatory forces than the trunk-conical morse cone.

This allowed us to start the systematic search of the most suitable rotation centre for each patient.

Another advantage of the modular neck is the possibility of removing it by means of the appropriate instruments set in case of cup revision thus allowing an excellent visibility of the acetabulum.

As for cups the exigency of modularity is certainly less important even though, in case of revision, the availability of hooks, rings or fins has resulted to be useful escpecially when bone graft is required.

In the first implants we used, as previously said, the ceramic-ceramic coupling, because all studies show that the use of polyethylene causes debriding, responsible for the osteholisis which leads to the loosening of the implant.

Also the metal-metal coupling has led to an even larger debris release and shown a lower biocompatibility than the ceramic-ceramic which is therefore, in our opinion, the most advantageous coupling.

The ceramics used in these couplings is alumina (alumina oxyde, Al_2O_3).

This material, besides the excellent biocompatibility, the absence of toxicity and mutagenicity, does not present any degradation.

Thanks to its surface it has a very low friction and is resistant to wear and rigid.

On the other hand the disadvantages of such coupling are implied in the characteristics of ceramics.

The criticisms initially raised against the ceramic-ceramic coupling were based upon the conviction that the rigidity in load transmission, the possibility of an incorrect positioning of the acetabulum or stem led to the possibility of a serious wear of ceramics with consequent failure of the implant.

Such disadvantage was clear in the implants where the alumina cup was cemented. The rigid load transmission entailed the break of the cement and consequently an anomalous ceramic-ceramic contact due to the cup instability.

The present assembly of ceramics in titanium metal-back and the use of press fit avoids this complication. When we used threaded cups where an important primary stability had to be found through the reaming of the acetabulum, we had to retain as much subcondral bone as possible.

Presently with press fit cups the stabilisation is no longer so important as the bone ingrowth must be reached in a short time. When implanting these cups, therefore, a particular care must be paid to expose as much bleeding cancellous bone as possible in order to get the osteointegration in a short time.

The implant of a press fit cup in a sclerotic and not bleeding bone will easily lead to an absence of bone ingrowth and a successive instability of the cup.

Another precaution we use during our ceramic-ceramic implant is that of avoiding the use of fixation screws in the cups.

Moreover the press fit uncemented cups reduce positioning mistakes as it is possible to correct the inclination of the cup during the implant phase (which was impossible with threaded cups).

Results

325 were recontrolled with a minimum follow up of 24 months (max 63 months), by carrying out outpatient, clinical and x-rays controls at 3rd, 6th, 12th month and afterwards every year.

Our surgical technique envisages a lateral transgluteal approach according to Bauer which allows a rapid access to the joint and an excellent visibility.

All the patients did not load the limb operated on for about 25 days after the surgery.

The functional clinical evaluation according to Harris showed good or excellent results with average values higher than 80 points, also considering the young age of the patients treated; also from the x-rays point of view the results were encouraging (though the survey and follow up were short). We have evaluated the correct orientation of the cup and stem, their possible mobilization, the possible presence of periprosthetic calcification.

In all the cases the orientation of the cup resulted to be satisfactory, there were no cases of prosthetic luxation, neither lines of radioshine nor osteolithic areas were found in the stem and cup area, on the contrary both resulted to be perfectly osteointegrated.

Pitfalls

The only problem which rose with the ceramic-ceramic coupling was the break of the ceramic inlay of a cup in a young patient (46 years) suffering from coxarthrosis in hip dysplasia. The incorrect positioning of the inlay in the metal-back caused an inaccurate alignment of the former and after few days of loading of the limb caused the break of the inlay.

The inlay was easily replaced.

Amongst our failures there were also two precocious infections of the implant. They were treated with specific antibiotic therapy and successively the implants were performed again.

At the beginning of our survey we had some problems due to the rigidity of the implant caused by the formation of several periarticular calcifications. The problem was solved through the administration of Indometacina 100mg suppositories for 8 days starting from the day of the surgery. In the cases regarded as riskier we used with excellent results a pre-operative cobalt therapy session (one hour before the surgery).

Bibliography

1. Dorre E.: Processing, Properties and Application of alumina implants. Biomaterials 1989.
2. Toni A. et al.: La ceramica nella chirurgia protesica dell'anca. Stato dell'arte. La Chirurgia degli Organi di Movimento. Vol. LXXX, 1995.
3. Rosner B.I., Postak P.D., Seth Greenwald A.: Cup/Liner Incongruity of two piece acetabular design: implications in the generation of Polyethylene debris. AAOS, 1994.
4. Puhl, W. (ed.): Bioceramics in Orthopaedics, New Applications, Enke, Stuttgart, 1998.
5. Ravaglioli A., Krajewsky A.: Bioceramics-Materials, Properties, Applications. Chapman and Hall, London, 1992.
6. Black J.: Biological Performance of Materials – Foundamentals of biocompatibility, Marcel Dekker, Inc., New York, 1992.
7. Sedel L. et al., Alumina-Alumina hip replacement in patients younger than 50 years old, Clin. Ortho. Rel. Res. 298 (1994) 175–183.
8. Puhl, W. (ed): Performance of the wear couple BIOLOX forte in hip arthroplasty. Enke. Stuttgart, 1997.

1.5 From Ceramics to Ceramics. Revisions of THR

J. Fenollosa, J. Baeza-Noci, P. Seminario

The use of a hard couple in total hip replacements intents to bypass the certain onset of failure caused by the polyethylene wear in the soft metal and ceramic-UHMWPE couples. Even with the hard bearings failure can arrive early in the first postoperative year, because of complications such as dislocation or sepsis and lately by loosening of the femoral or acetabular pieces, once surpassed the eight to ten year mark. We have analysed our cases of failure in order to determine the avoidable cases and the possibility of treatment once they appear, saving the long-term durability of the alumina couple.

We have used two types of modular THR as carriers of an alumina ceramic couple. The first nine years 1981- 1990 we employed the cemented stem and cemented ceramic cup or the cemented stem self threading metal back cup manufactured by Ceraver under the trade mark Osteal with 32 mm diameter heads. The last nine years 1990 – 1998 we have used press fit cups with cementless stems, a few Ceraver Cerafit with 32 mm head and the majority manufactured by LIMA LTO under the trade name F2L- SPH with 28 mm heads.

Our indication for use of the alumina ceramic couple has always been the long life expectancy of the patients. In our own cases the indication has been firstly as a primary operation, secondly in those operated elsewhere as the hardware used in revision surgery to correct the use of failed prostheses with metal – PE couples, in patients under sixty five years of age.

The complications of our own ceramic prostheses leading to its replacement have been mainly of two types: mechanical or biologic. Mechanical complications are those menacing or impeding the correct function of the couple, they appear in the postoperative period of days or weeks after the primary operation. The most frequent is the excessive verticality of the cup that leads ineluctably to wear in the ridge of contact. The insufficient anteversion of the cup and retroversion of the neck leads also to failures: the spontaneous dislocation of the hip. In a few cases the interface between the metal cup and the ceramic insert can jam. Of similar type but later onset is the impingement of neck against cup in the skirted heads or thick metal necks than can produce recurrent dislocation or wearing. In the cases of surgical revision of previous ceramic couples the mismatch of types of cone of head and stem can lead to broken head, early metal wear or late fretting corrosion (1, 4, 16, 19).

Biological complications are the sepsis, the heterotopic bone formation and the aseptic loosening of cup or stem. The sepsis appears as different clinical settings, Gustilo classified them in four types: early in the immediate postoperative period even with wound closed or late chronic even years after primary hip replacement, consequence of the operative contamination or hematogenous colonisation. We will not examine here the last clinical setting of infection, says the positive culture in revisions (14, 18).

The heterotopic bone formation was classed by Brooker and al in four types, they are universally used and as that have been applied in our cases of THR (3).

The loosening of prostheses is a tardive complication and has been the object of numberless articles. It appears mostly after the eighth year in cups and the twelfth year in stems. The causes are multiple, related to the appearance of fibrous membranes in the interfaces between cement metal and bone, and for the most caused by a mechanical failure that can be started by the particles illness described by Willert. The latest complication is the osteolysis either of femur or acetabulum, or unfortunately in too many cases in both places (17).

We have suffered the whole catalogue of problems, in the three types of ceramic bearing prostheses we have used cemented, hybrid or cementless, but the frequency is different and of diverse importance according to the type. Let examine them more closely.

We have used to the time of this writing the alumina ceramic bearing in 121 all cemented and 41 hybrid prostheses, 73 of them in patients under 50 years being reported to the SOFCOT Congress in 1997. 257 cementless prostheses with 85 patients of less than 50 years of age were treated in the years 1990 to 1998. All the femoral prostheses and the metal back cups were of TiVAl alloy. The hybrid prostheses had the metal back cup brightly polished and the cementless THR have both stem and cup of rough surface partially covered by osteoconductive material. The bearing was of 32-mm diameter until 1993 and of 28 mm afterward. All the prostheses were operated by a team of different surgeons in the same unit of a teaching hospital by posterolateral approach (8).

Complications and Failures

All Cemented Prostheses

In those THR we suffered five early failures: two fractures of the diaphysis of the femur one of them leading to a perioperative death while being treated by internal fixation with a plate, the other leading to an early revision at the eleventh month for persistent pain at the thigh. One vertical cup that was changed to a normal position at the 7th month, fearing quick wear. One sepsis with open sinuses appeared at the seventh month, a salmonella typhi was cultured in them and the patient was treated successfully by a two step revision, with secondary insertion of the same type of prosthesis using antibiotic cement. One of the postoperative luxations was reduced by open reduction and not recurred.

Although not causing immediate failure we observed in the first postoperative X-ray in some cases lateral flares of cement, extruded through longitudinal fissures of the shaft of the femur. We believe this fact is due, as the perioperative fractures, to the limited range of femoral broaches of this particular type of cemented prostheses. The increase in rasp size is not regularly progressive; their use may open longitudinally the diaphysis if the rasping is prosecuted too energetically searching a tightly seated prosthesis.

As late complications we have suffered in the all cemented THR, one infection by Staphylococcus Aureus appearing at the 46th month spontaneously, treated by a Girdlestone arthroplasty and causing nonetheless the exitus of the patient by septicaemia. One fracture of a ceramic head needing surgical revision, careful culling of fragments jet lavage and synovectomy. Heterotopic bone was seen infrequently in these prostheses, classed by the Brooker system we found: one case of types II and four cases of type IV. (1, 6, 3).

The quality of cementing was classed after Barrack: in the femur we obtained 21% of type A, 50% type B, 27% type C and 2% type D. We classed the bone defects in those loose THR according to Paprosky. We found in the femur: one case of type 1, ten cases of 2 A and two cases of 2 B. As to the acetabulum we found: two cases of 2 A, five cases of 2B, two cases of 2C, two of 3 A and three cases of 3B types. Sixteen patients suffered loosening of their prostheses, we followed the Harris system of definite, probable and possible failures. We operated them in cases of continuous pain in any of the three radiological classes. So we found 5 failures of a single component: 3 cases of loose cup and 2 of loose stem; 2 cases suffered a progressive failure first of the stem and then of the cup and 9 cases a double simultaneous failure of both com-

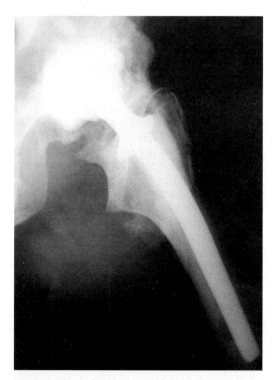

Fig. 1 Cemented ceramic prosthesis showing an intracortical cyst in zone V

ponents. The mean time of failure was of 8.3 years (2 – 17 yr. range). The loose THR have been treated mainly by big bore cementless prostheses and cups (all but eight cases at the beginning of our experience, for that more will be told later) supported by morselized allografts in acetabulum and milled bone in femur respectively. The new stem was 10 times a LCR Lima, 2 times a F2L also from Lima, 1 a Profile and 1 a Solution prosthesis from De Puy. The cup 10 times a SPH Lima with six ceramic and 4 PE inserts, 1 Profile De Puy and 1 Octofit Tornier with PE liner and 1 cemented all PE cup. The remaining was one bipolar head. From a preoperative 1-3-3 D'Aubigné score they reached 5.3 – 5.3 – 4.7 in pain, mobility and march after surgical revision. The bone defects due to osteolysis were observed only in the cases of loose components and localized according to De Lee for acetabulum and Gruen for femur. Only one case of intracortical cystic lysis was observed in a well-fixed femur in zone V. This THR suffered a loose cup with acetabular osteolysis, we couldn't ascertain if due to ceramic or PMMA particles despite a microscopic examination of a punch specimen (8, 13, 15) (Figure 1).

Hybrid Prostheses

These THR as well as the all cemented prostheses with 32-mm alumina couple are of Osteal manufacture. The stem has a rectangular section of Ti-VAl, the junction between head and neck by Morse taper, the cup a TiVAl troncoconical self-threading flat top, with conical polished inside and outside to a mirror finish, with an alumina liner of outer non polished surface and conical section.

We suffered five early complications leading in one case of perioperative type III femoral fracture to a simultaneous ORIF by plate and periprosthetic screws. The cause of this fracture has been referred already as due to an excessively simple ancillary. The other four complications needed a secondary surgical revision. Two vertical cups were observed in the postoperative X-ray and were reoperated in the days following the primary surgery to correct the position to a 45° abduction + 10° anteversion angle. One patient suffered an accident at the third month losing the grip of the cup into the bone and dislocating the whole metal-liner component. One patient suffered the jamming of the alumina liner in an ex-centred position with the chamber of the metal cup; it went undetected for ten months until it gripped. All the four early failing self-threading metal cups were surgically changed to cemented alumina couples of the same manufacturer without need for bone graft. The cemented stem showed a Barrack's cement mantle of quality A in 52%, B in 33% and C in 15% of the cases. This type of prosthesis showed a high frequency of heterotopic ossification with one Brooker type I, none type II, six type III and one type IV (Figure 2).

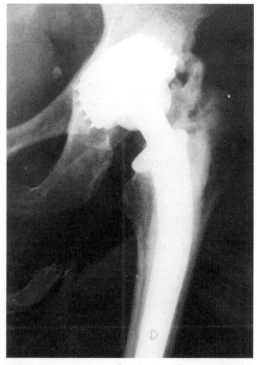

Fig. 2 Heterotopic ossification Brooker IV around a self-threaded metal cup

We suffered one deep sepsis with positive culture to akinetobacter calcoacetii and one superficial wet wound with positive culture to Staphylococcus epidermis. The deep sepsis was treated by a two step revision with intermediate gentamycin beads filling (18).

The hybrid prostheses loosened in 8 of 41 cases (19%) in patients of 65 years of mean age, range 54 – 73 years. Those cups failed at 7 years of mean life, 2 – 11 years of range. The failures were one only of the cup, the cup first then the stem in one case, the stem first then the cup one case and both together four cases. The stem failure showed a strong relation with the quality of the cement mantle: no loose stem if the quality was A, 23% of failures in B quality and 15% of failures if C quality. Pain plus migration of more than 4 mm or 5° rotation signed for us the failures of the cup. The bone defects as of Paprosky were in the femur six times of 2 A and one 2 B, in the acetabulum one case of 2 B, one of 2C, three times 3 A and 3 times 3C. Those grave bone defects asked for bone allograft in all cases of revision and one Burch-Schneider ring in a 3C defect. The material employed in the revision was four times one LCR and three F2L stems all of Lima manufacture. The cups were six big bore SPH Lima with alumina liner in patients under seventy. One De Puy Profile with PE liner and one all PE cup cemented over the Burch ring. The Merle D'Aubigné score went from 1-3-4 preoperatively to 6-6-6 postoperatively. It is interesting to note the good clinical results after revision of the hybrid prostheses, that we ascribe to an early treatment and the absence of PMMA or UHMWPE in the acetabulum, even with cases of transgression of the medial wall by the metallic cup. This type of cup has been abandoned by the promoters of the technique for the same cause than us, namely the high percentage of failures. We continue to use the hybrid prostheses in cases of femur with a cortical relation higher than 75% but with press fit hemispherical cup and cobalt-chrome collared stem (15).

Revisions using the Alumina Cemented or Hybrid Prostheses

This technique was used in our Unit with uniformly bad results in eight cases. We abandoned it in 1989. They were cases of relatively young patients, 60 years of mean age, bearers of three Müller cemented „banana" type with 32 mm couple metal polyethylene, two Charnley LFA 22 mm and one cementless PM of 32 mm metal-UHMWPE couple prostheses. The initial diagnoses were four O.A., one sequel of B. Koch arthritis, one dysplastic hip sequel of polio, time to failure 38 months. Two more cases were of femoral prostheses after a neck fracture, with a Müller Trilock modular and a Thompson both of metal head prostheses. They passed from a score of 1-5.5 – 2 preoperatively to 3.5 – 5.5 – 3.5 postoperatively. Notwithstanding the use of bone grafts in 100% of the cases we suffered two perioperative fractures and later on loosening of four stems and four cups. The preoperative state of bone stock was in the femur: two Paprosky's type 1, one case of 2 A and two type 3 lesions. In the acetabulum the bone loss was one type 1, one 2 A, one 2 C and two cases of 3 A lesions. In one of the cases of sequel of fracture the use of a ceramic head and a TiVAl neck of different manufacturer lead to an accelerated metal wear in six months. These shotgun marriages must be avoided at all cost (Figure 3).

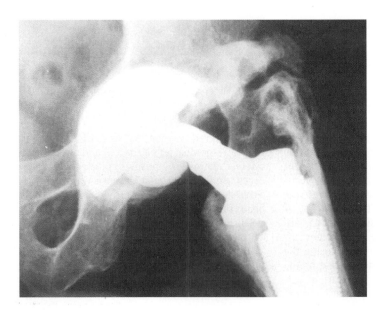

Fig. 3 Accelerated wear of a TiVAl neck by a ceramic head of different manufacturer

Cementless Alumina Prostheses

This type of prostheses has been in use in our unit since 1990, first in 32-mm couple with a Titanium mesh covered cup „Cerafit" by Osteal. Later the great majority in 28 mm couple Biolox Forte under the trade name SPH cup and F2L modular stem and neck by Lima LTO.

In this particular type of prostheses we have suffered 13 failures, six early and seven late. The early failures requiring operation were of different types: one postoperative luxation, 1 jammed insert in the cup, two malposition: one cup and one stem respectively and two cases of deep sepsis of early onset before the 30th day. The late failures were two recurrent dislocations, two loosening of the stem, one vertical position leading to loosening of the cup and two loosening of cups with normal position. They affected two „Cerafit" titanium mesh covered cups and ten „SPH" HA covered cups in TiVAl. They have been all surgically revised and replaced by prostheses F2L of alumina bearing. We have suffered moreover seven postoperative luxations; they were treated by closed reduction under anaesthesia and remain asymptomatic until this writing so they are not included in the description.

Two early deep sepses were cultured and gave positive to staphylococcus Aureus and pseudomona aeruginosa. In both cases after a short course of the appropriate antibiotic as determined by the culture, the wound was surgically open before the 21tst day, layer by layer were excised as far as to arrive to sound normal looking tissue, in these early sepsis no sinuses were found. Once one layer was excised the wound was irrigated with 5‰ chlorhexidin solution, then the next layer open it was washed with pulsating jet lavage with one unit of saline serum. Then it was excised and irrigated anew with chlorehexidin, until the joint was reached. The prosthesis was dislocated, the alumina head and insert removed. When the metal pieces are well fixed as they were in these two cases, the metallic pieces were thoroughly washed with pulsating lavage and immersed for five minutes in clorhexidin. The draping and instruments changed a new neck head and insert were placed and temporary the wound closed over a suction drain per layer, gentamycin beads strings placed into the joint and in the subcutaneous fat layer, until the seventh day. The drains were removed once they became dry. Both cases have remained healed uneventfully two and three years later (14, 18).

One insert jammed in an asymmetrical position, the upper third of the circle sunk into the TiVAl cup, the inferior part blocked against the outside metal ridge, so as to have the metal cup in a 45° inclination position whilst the ceramic liner is in a more vertical position. It happened once in the Osteal self-threading cup and once in the SPH press-fit cup with bare ceramic liner of

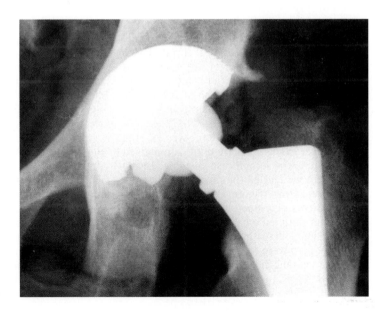

Fig. 4 Jammed ceramic liner into a metal back impacted cup

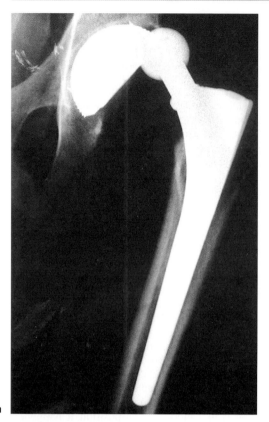 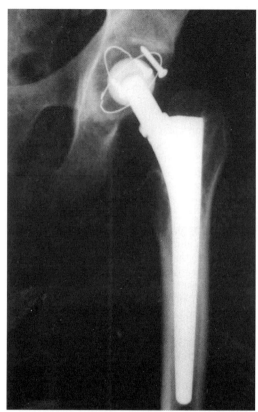

Fig. 5 Press-fit cementless THR a) showing hip luxation b) the same stem and head with a cemented PE socket and PE supplement fixed by screws

the first series, because the outside of the ceramic liner not so well polished as the inside blocked. In both cases the surgical approach was tight due to the difficulties of the case. It has never happened again since our using of the ceramic liner with an outside shell of GUR 15 PE that lubricates the entry into the metal cup. The postoperative X Ray made the day after the operation showed the malposition, we let the jammed liner in the first case until pain obliged to change it, in the second case knowing already the problem we revised the prosthesis once the malfunction known (Figure 4).

Two patients developed a recurrent luxation, one of them suffered on a unilateral OA and the other a bilateral idiopathic necrosis of the head of the femur. Both were revised, the unilateral case showed a ceramic ridge fractured and a black metallic tattoo in the site of the neck impingement. This case was treated by picking by hand the macroscopic fragments, complete synovectomy, abundant pulsated washing of the joint to remove the microscopic ceramic fragments than could lead to third body wear, change of both ceramic components after careful inspection and cleaning of the trunion and cup surfaces. The patient with the bilateral necrosis, the hip first treated ten years before by a well functioning cemented ceramic, the second hip with a press-fit F2L prosthesis developed a recurrent dislocation. He was treated by a first operation that changed the neck, putting a long one in order to increase the offset and tighten the muscles. This limited operation failed. He suffered a posterior luxation while abroad in holidays and was treated in another hospital, were the metal back cup was changed for a cemented all PE cup more anteversed. Returning home it dislocated anew; this time in an anterior position; we treated him by a third operation inserting a quarter melon

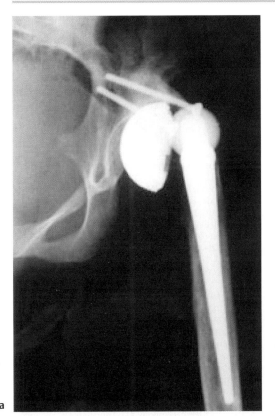 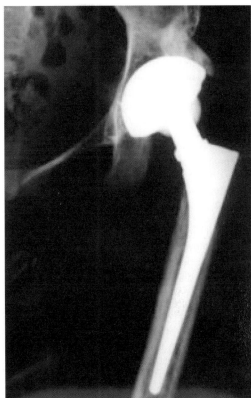

Fig. 6 Traumatic luxation of a F2L prosthesis on a dysplasic hip, bone shelf fixed by cortical stellite screws b) correction with a bigger cup deeply seated

polyethylene fixed forward to the previous cup by two stellite screws. It has remained asymptomatic since then, knowing of the possibility of an early wear. In the case of luxation we recommend the CAT of the hip, knee and ankle in order to know the relative acetabular and neck anteversion. All the abnormal position must be surgically corrected without waiting to new luxations to prevent the damage of the ceramic ridge by impingement. The neck of ceramic prostheses must not be of bigger dimensions than 12/14, the slimmer the better, in order to avoid the impingement in flexion external rotation. For the same reasons no skirted head must be allowed in hard bearings (5, 12) (Figure 5).

Four patients suffered loosening, two of them of the femur, appearing clinically as thigh pain with hot points to the isotopic scintigraphy and subsidence visible in the X Ray, they were treated by exchange to a bigger stem of the same type over a bone allograft filling with good results. Two cups suffered a mobilisation. A Cerafit of titanium mesh cover was placed in near 90° inclination fixed with an auxiliary screw. The patient developed pain after six years. The faulty cup was revised and changed to a new press-fit cup of bigger diameter HA covered. She has remained with a 6-6-6 score since, with two years of follow up. The second failed cup suffered a progressive loosening, it was a hemispherical mesh covered cup fixed by two screws proximally. Moreover one SPH cup in a severe dysplasic hip of Crowe III type, suffered a fall two years after her first operation. The prosthesis dislocated and the cup mobilized. Deepening the socket bed and taking out the screws fixing the bone shelf of the primary operation repaired this case. Then we changed to a bigger cup of the same type. The cup retired showed a 15% of the surface with bone ingrowth and no HA remaining in the rough TiVAl surface (2, 11, 14) (Figure 6).

Conclusions

We have improved our results, by two reasons, first the improving of the materials, ceramics of smaller grain and increased density. Second the changes of our own surgical technique, avoiding capsulectomy and keeping the piriformis tendon preserved for a better tenure of the prosthesis inside the articular cavity to prevent dislocation. Dislocation can be harmful to the ceramic liner, breaking or tattooing it and must not be allowed to repeat.

We don't use anymore cement as a fixation device. Cementless prostheses have allowed us to safeguard the bone stock, even in cases of loosening. The use of HA covered cup and stem has diminished the loosening in the series where it has been employed. Our own series follows this tendency. The early treatment of sepsis is another factor avoiding the bone loss.

The presence of a PE layer over the ceramic has solved the quite specific complication of the ceramic alumina couple in metal cup: the jammed liner. The cases of unexplained pain should be revised early, even if the cause is not visible at x-rays: a loose prosthesis is to be expected in the presence of pain. The use of a modular neck has permitted us to change neck and ceramic head without touching the stem, avoiding in cases of revision thus a dangerous step. In revisions the compacted milled allograft with bigger press-fit acetabular cups seems to be a technique as satisfactory in the cementless prostheses as in the cemented ones (11).

Bibliography

1. Allain J, Goutallier D, Voisin MC, Lemouel S.: Failure of a stainless-steel femoral head of a revision total hip arthroplasty performed after a fracture of a ceramic femoral head. J Bone Joint Surg 80 A, 1355–1360, 1998
2. Bloebaum RD, Jensen JW, Dorr LD: Post-mortem analysis of bone ingrowth into porous-coated acetabular components. J Bone Joint Surg 1997, 79, 1013–1022
3. Brooker AF, Bowerman JW, Robinson RA, Riley LH: Ectopic ossification following total hip replacement Incidence and a method of classification. J Bone Joint Surg, 55 A, 1629–1632, 1973
4. Collier JP, Mayor MB, Jensen RE, et al.: Mechanism of failure of modern prostheses. Clin Orthop 285, 129–140, 1992
5. Daly PJ, Morrey BF: Operative correction of an unstable total hip arthroplasty. J Bone Joint Surg 1992. 74 A, 1334–1343
6. Dorr L, Zhinian W.: Causes and treatment protocol for instability of total hip replacement. Clin Orthop 355, 144–151, 1998
7. Engh CA, Hooten JP, Zetti-Schaffer KF: Evaluation of bone ingrowth in proximally and extensively porous-coated anatomic medullary locking prostheses retrieved at autopsy. J Bone Joint Surg, 1995, 77 A, 903–910
8. Fenollosa J. Aparisi JM, Seminario P: Résultats à long terme des prothèses de hanche alumine-alumine. Rev. Chir. Orthop 83. Supplement II, 44, 1997
9. Fritsch EW, Gleitz M.: Ceramic femoral head fractures in total hip arthroplasty. Clinical Orthop, 1996, 328, 129–136
10. Gie GA, Linder L, Ling RSM, Simon JF, Sloof TJJH, Timperley AJ: Impacted cancellous allografts and cement for revision total hip arthroplasty. J Bone Joint Surg 1993, 75B, 14–21.
11. Gristina AG, Costerton JW: Bacterial adherence to biomaterials and tissue, The significance of its role in clinical sepsis. J Bone Joint Surg. 67 A, 264–273, 1985
12. Huten D: Luxations et subluxations des prothèses totales de hanche. Cahiers d'Enseignement SOFCOT, Conférences d'Enseignement 1996, 19–46, 1996
13. Merle D'Aubigné R. Postel M: Functional results of hip arthroplasty with acrylic prostheses. J Bone Joint Surg, 36 A: 451–475, 1954
14. Pagnano MW, Hanssen AD, Lewallen DG, Shaughnessy WJ: The effect of superior placement of the acetabular component and the rate of loosening after total hip arthroplasty. J.Bone Joint Surg. 78 A, 1004–1014. 1996
15. Paprosky W, Lawrence J, Cameron H: Acetabular defect classification: clinical application. Orthop Rev. 19 (Supplement 9): 3–9, 1990. Femoral defect classification: clinical application. Ortop Rev. 19 (Supplement 9): 9–15, 1990
16. Peiro A, Pardo J, Navarrete R, Rodriguez Alonso L, Martos F.: Fracture of the ceramic head in total hip arthroplasty, Report of two cases. J Arthroplasty 6: 371–374, 1991
17. Taek Rim Yoon, Sung Man Rowe, Sung Taek Jung, Kwang Jin Seon, Maloney WJ: Osteolysis in association with a total hip arthroplasty with ceramic bearing surfaces. J Bone Joint Surg, 80 A, 1459–1468, 19
18. Tsukayama DT, Estrada R, Gustilo R.: Infection after total hip arthroplasty. A study of the treatment of one hundred and six infections. J Bone Joint Surg, 78 A. 512–523, 1996

1.6 Analyse unserer Erfahrungen mit Keramik/Keramik-Hüftendoprothesen der ersten Generation (1974–1978)

P. Griss, A. Claus und G. Scheller

Die LINDENHOF-Endoprothese mit Keramikschraubpfanne, Keramikkugelkopf und zementiertem Schaft war das erste in Deutschland eingesetzte Kunstgelenk dieser Materialkombination (5; Abb. 1). Sie wurde am 26.9.1974 erstmals implantiert. Zuvor war diese Gleitpaarung in Hybridtechnik allerdings bereits 1970 von P. Boutin in Frankreich inauguriert worden (1, 2, 3). In Mannheim wurden bis zum 4.10.1978 insgesamt 97 Lindenhofprothesen bei 84 Patienten verwendet. Eine erste mittelfristige Analyse zeigte bereits die materialspezifischen Probleme (6, 9), die in einer späteren Auswertung 10–12 Jahre post-op. erneut aktualisiert dokumentiert wurden (14) und uns damals veranlaßt haben, diese Prothese nicht mehr zu verwenden.

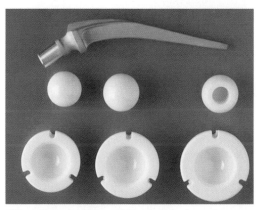

Abb. 1 Lindenhof-Keramik/Keramik-Endoprothese, Pfanne zementfrei, Schaft immer zementiert.

Inzwischen ist die Entwicklung klinisch weitergegangen, der Polyaethylenabrieb hat sich zu einem zentralen Langzeitproblem für die Haltbarkeit der Endoprothese entwickelt, neue abriebarme und im Abrieb bioreaktionsarme Lösungen werden gefördert bzw. leben mit verbesserter Technologie wieder auf (Metall/Metall, Keramik/Keramik, Keramik/ vernetztes Polyaethylen; 13,

15). Die derzeitige Qualität der Al_2O_3-Keramik bietet nun bessere Lösungen und Langzeitaussichten für Hüftgelenkkonstruktionen als dies mit der von uns damals verwendeten Keramik möglich war.

Da das Material aber unverändert spröde und extrem hart ist, gelten heute wie damals grundsätzlich gleiche Regeln und Grenzen der Keramikanwendung im Hüftbereich freilich derzeit mit deutlich höherem Sicherheitsniveau. Die Gesetze der Bruchmechanik sind unverändert limitierend, Abrieb bei linearer Belastung ist weiter zu erwarten, Abriebpartikel können unverändert gefährlich werden sowohl als Dreikörperverschleißkomponente als auch biologisch über Makrophagenreaktionen (7, 8, 11, 12). Die Analyse der ersten Generation von Keramik/Keramik-Endoprothesen, vor allem jetzt nach 21–25 Jahren kann uns helfen alte Fehler zu vermeiden und neue besser zu verstehen.

Im Herbst 1998 haben A.C. und G.S. das Mannheimer Krankengut erneut ausgewertet. Tabelle 1 berichtet über den aktuellen Stand.

Tabelle 1 Aktueller Stand Lindenhof-Endoprothesen

N = 97 Prothesen bei 84 Patienten
35 Patienten mit 37 Prothesen reoperiert (36%)
16 Patienten verstorben (15%)
14 Patienten nicht mehr auffindbar (13%)
23 Pat. mit 25 Prothesen noch in situ (24%)

Von der letzen Gruppe in Tab. 1 konnten 19 Patienten mit 21 Prothesen klinisch und radiologisch nachuntersucht werden. Zunächst jedoch die Analyse der reoperierten Fälle. Tab. 2 gibt hierzu Auskunft.

Tab. 3 unterrichtet über die Zeitabläufe bis zur Reoperation. Interessant und nur schwer zu interpretieren sind die grossen Zeitspannen bei den Keramikkopfbrüchen und den Pfannenwanderungen. Letztere können nach Einzelbeobachtungen noch nach mehr als 20 Jahren dokumentiert

Tabelle 2 Aktueller Stand Lindenhof-Endoprothesen, Indikation zur Reoperation

N = 37 Prothesen bei 35 Patienten (36% d. Gesamtkollektivs)	
Keramikkopfbruch	9 (8,7%)
Pfannenlockerung und Migration	12 (11,6%)
Pfannen- und Schaftlockerung	12 (11,6%)
Tiefe Infektion	2 (1,9%)
Prothesenschaftbruch	2 (1,9%)

Tabelle 3 Darstellung der Zeitabläufe bis zur Reoperation

Keramikkopfbruch	3 Mo–10J/6Mo
Pfannenwanderung	3J/10 Mo–21 J
Pfannen- und Schaftlockerung	1J/6 Mo–18 J
Sept. Lockerung	20 Mo und 49 Mo
Prothesenschaftbruch (gl. Pat. bds.)	53 Mo und 64 Mo

idealem Sitz der Pfanne unvermittelt beginnen und dann innerhalb eines Jahres schnell fortschreiten. Hier spielt offenbar spät einsetzender Dreikörperverschleiß mit exponentiell ansteigenden Abriebvolumina die entscheidende Rolle (siehe unser zweiter Beitrag in diesem Symposium).

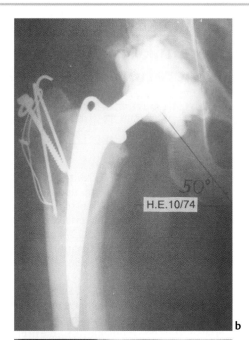

b

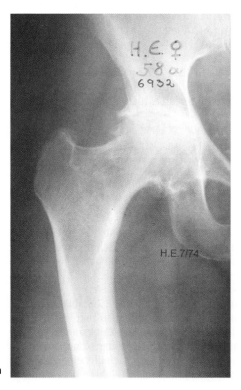

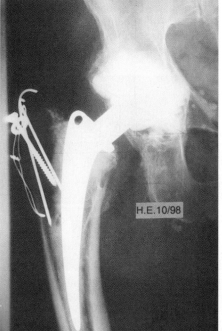

c

Abb. 2a–c Pat. H.E. (erster operierter Fall).
a) Rö.A. rechte Hüfte a.p. praeoperativ.
b) Direkt postoperative Rö.A. 1974 der rechten Hüfte.
c) Letzte Rö.A. 1999, 25 Jahre postoperativ. Die Pfanne hat sich etwas flacher gestellt und ist um 2mm nach zentral gewandert, zementierter Schaft unverändert, keine Osteolysen.

Die Auswertung von 21 nachuntersuchten Prothesen bei 19 Patienten (21–25 Jahre post-op.) zeigt erstaunliche Verläufe und Einzelbeobachtungen. 16 Patienten sind völlig beschwerdefrei und gehfähig (HARRIS hip score: 65–100 Punkte, Mittel 84,6), 5 Patienten berichten über Beschwerden beim Gehen. Die radiologische Auswertung bestätigt erneut, daß Klinik und Röntgenbildanalyse nicht zuverlässig korrelieren. Die Pfannenwanderung war auch hier wesentliches quantitativ erfaßbares Spätproblem. Sie wurde in drei Kategorien eingeteilt. Bei 4 Pfannen in Gruppe 1 (Migration <= 2 mm) fehlten klinische Zeichen, weder Säume noch Osteolysen noch Dezentrierung des Kopfes waren feststellbar (Abb.2). 7 Pfannen in Gruppe 2 (Migration 3–10 mm) zeigten Wanderung nach zentral und kranial, wobei das Implantat sich sowohl flacher (5x) als auch zusätzlich steiler (1x) einstellen konnte. Ein Fall zeigte dabei Schaftosteolysen, in einem Fall war der Schaft um 5 mm eingesunken. Die Patientin mit der Schaftosteolyse hatte als Einzige klinisch Beschwerden. Bei 10 Pfannen der Gruppe 3 war eine Wanderung von mehr als 10 mm nachweisbar. Hier waren 4 Patienten klinisch auffällig (1x Pfannenlockerung und Schaftosteolyse, 1x Schaft eingesunken; Abb. 3).

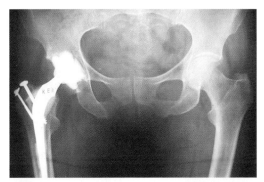

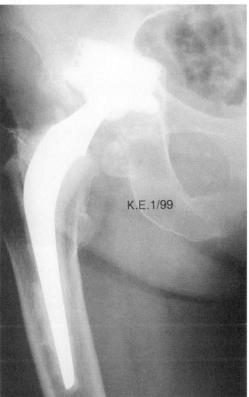

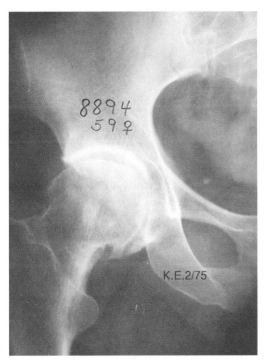

Abb. 3a–c Pat. K.E., operiert 2, 1975.
a) Praeop. Rö.A. rechte Hüfte a.p.
b) Beckenübersicht 8 Monate postoperativ, regulärer Sitz der Implantate.
c) Rö.A. der rechten Hüfte 24 Jahre postoperativ, Kippung und massive Kranial- bzw. Zentralwanderung der Pfanne, keinerlei Schaftosteolysezeichen.

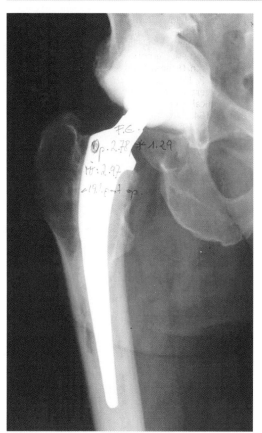

Faßt man die Analyse der Schadensfälle und die Befunde der Nachuntersuchung zusammen, so war es richtig 1978 die weitere Implantation dieser Prothese zu stoppen. Langzeitberichte über Keramik/Keramik-Endoprothesen der ersten Generation anderer Hersteller und Konstruktion bestätigen unsere Befunde (4, 10, 16). Läßt man die Kopfbrüche außer Acht, so ist die Pfannenwanderung und Lockerung das wesentliche, nach 21–25 Jahren von einzelnen Ausnahmen abgesehen (Abb. 4) bei der Mehrzahl der Prothesen in situ nachweisbare, die Lebenszeit des Kunstgelenkes limitierende Phänomen. Alle bisher reoperierten Implantate zeigen z.T. erhebliche Substanzverluste durch Abrieb. Interessanterweise scheint hier die Ausgangsposition der Pfanne nicht entscheidend zu sein, da sowohl bei zentral, oder in varus oder valgus gekippten Pfannen stets deutliche Abriebverluste festzustellen waren. Je mehr gewandert, desto mehr Abrieb scheint die Erfahrung zu zeigen. Wir vermuten deshalb, daß mit der Zunahme der Pfannenwanderung und so zunehmend breiter werdendem Verschleißspalt und Inkongruenz der Dreikörperverschleiss unter Einklemmung von Keramikabriebpartikeln die Rolle des exponentiell wachsenden Verschleißpromotors übernehmen kann (11, 12).

Dann finden sich auch in Einzelfällen z.T. ausgedehnte Osteolysen am Adamschen Bogen und tie-

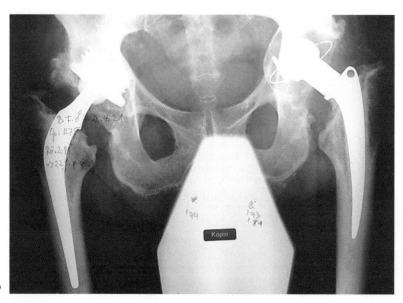

Abb. 4a,b Zwei Beispiele für gute Langzeitergebnisse.
a) Pat. F.G. Rö.A. rechte Hüfte a.p. 19 Jahre postoperativ; unveränderter Sitz der Implantate, der Pfannenboden war bei der Operation mit einer Spongiosascheibe aus dem Hüftkopf verstärkt worden.
b) Pat. B.F. Rö.A. Beckenübersicht rechts 22 Jahre post impl. Unveränderter Sitz der Implantate, links Wanderung einer gut 10 Jahre später eingesetzten Morscher-Pfanne.

fer an der Zement-Knochengrenze. Wie in unserer zweiten Mitteilung in diesem Symposium noch zu zeigen sein wird, können die Keramikabriebpartikel den Metallhals der Schaftprothese polieren und zerkratzen mit nachfolgender erheblicher Metallose und einem typischen Mischgranulom, das zusätzlich die Pfannen- und Schaftlockerung fördert. Korundpulver ist ein Standardmaterial für die Oberflächenbearbeitung von Metallen. Letztlich also dürften im Spätverlauf uniforme biologische Reaktionen zu erwarten sein, die stark von der Menge und der Grösse des Keramikabriebs und des ev. Sekundär entstehenden Metallabriebes diktiert werden. Es wird noch zu beweisen sein, ob die technisch optimierte Keramik, sowie die neuen Verankerungstechnologien (Titanring oder Schale mit Keramikinlay) die mechanisch einen ähnlich starren Verbund darstellen wie die alten Keramikendoprothesen den Test der Zeit im Patienten (nach 15 und mehr Jahren) bestehen. Trotz der Fortschritte bleiben die alten Erkenntnisse aus dieser Nachuntersuchung der heutigen Keramik verwandt. Sobald die Keramik die Produktionsstätte verlassen hat gelangt sie in die Hände des Operateurs und dann in den Körper des Patienten. Beides ist verbunden mit individuellen, die relativ enge Toleranzbreite der Keramik damals wie heute gefährdenden Unwägbarkeiten, die die Keramik/Keramik-Kombination auch in Zukunft auf die Probe stellen werden (13).

Literaturhinweise

1 Boutin, P. (1971): L'Alumine et son utilisation en chirurgie de la hange (Etude experimentale). Presse Med. 79, 639.
2 Boutin, P. (1972): Arthroplastie totale de la hange par prothese en alumine frittée. Revue Chir. Orthop. 58, 229–246.
3 Boutin, P., Christel, P., Dorlot, J.M., Meunier, A., de Roquancourt, A., Blanquaert, D., Herman, S., Sedel, L., Wivoet, J. (1988): The use of dense alumina-alumina ceramic combination in total hip replacement. J. Biomed. Mater. Res. 22, 1203–1232.
4 Garcia-Cimbrelo, E., Martinez-Sayanes, J.M., Mimisa, A., Munera, L.C. (1996): Mittelmeier ceramic-ceramic prosthesis after 10 years. J. Arthroplasty 11, 773–781.
5 Griss, P., Heimke, G., von Andrian- Werburg, H. F. (1975): Die Aluminiumoxidkeramik-Metall-Verbundendoprothese. Eine neue Hüftgelenks-Totalendoprothese zur teilweise zementfreien Implantation. Arch. Orthrop, Unfall-Chir. 81, 259–266.
6 Griss, P., Heimke, G. (1981): Five years experience with ceramic-metal-composite hip endoprostheses. I. Clinical evaluation. Arch. Orthop. Trauma Surg. 98, 157–164.
7 Griss, P. (1983): Ergebnisse der teilweise zementfrei implantierten Hüftendoprothese Typ Lindenhof 4–8 Jahre post operationem. In: E. Morscher, Die zementlose Fixation von Hüftendoprothesen. Springer-Verlag Berlin, Heidelberg pp. 226–230.
8 Griss, P., Hartz, U., Willert, H.-G. (1985): Analyse der periprothetischen Gewebereaktion bei 26 reoperierten Hüftendoprothesen der Al_2O_3-Keramik-Gleitpaarung. Z. Orthop. 123, 668–669.
9 Heimke, G., Griss, P. (1981): Five years experience with ceramic-metal-composite hip endoprostheses. II. Mechanical evaluations and improvements. Arch. Orthop. Trauma Surg. 98, 165–171.
10 Hyder, N., Nevelos, A.B., Barabas T.G. (1996): Cementless ceramic hip arthroplasties in patients less than 30 years old. J. Arthroplasty 11, 679–686.
11 Plitz, W., Griss, P. (1981): Clinical, histomorphological and material – related observations on removed alumina-ceramic hip joint components. Conf. Proc.: Implant retrieval: Material and biological aspects. Gaithersburg MD. 1980, U.S. Dept. Of Commerce pp. 131–147.
12 Plitz, W., Walter, A., Jäger, M. (1984): Materialspezific wear of ceramic/ceramic sliding surfaces in revised hip endoprostheses. Clinical and technological considerations. Z. Orthop. 122, 299–303.
13 Willmann, G. (1998): Ceramics for total hip replacement – what a surgeon should know. Orthopaedics 21, 173–177.
14 Winter, M., Griss, P., Scheller, G., Moser, T. (1992): Ten – to 14 – year results of a ceramic hip prosthesis. Clin. Orthop. 282, 73–80.
15 Wroblewski, B.M., Siney, P.D., Dowson, D., Collins, S.N. (1996): Prospective clinical and joint simulator studies of a new total hip arthroplasty using alumina ceramic heads and cross-linked polyaethylene cups. J. Bone Jt. Surg. 78B, 280–285.
16 Yoon, T.R., Rowe, S.M., Jung, S.T., Seon, K.J., Maloney, W.J. (1998): Osteolysis in association with a total hip arthroplasty with ceramic bearing surfaces. J.Bone Jt. Surg. 80A, 1459–1468.

1.7 6-Jahres-Ergebnisse des Axis-Hüftendoprothesensystems, basierend auf 25 Jahren Erfahrung mit Aluminiumoxydhartgleitpaarungen

B. Schuhmacher, H. Beck, D. Stock

Die jahrelang anscheinend problemlose endoprothetische Versorgung unzähliger Hüftpatienten war ein wesentlicher Grund für die weltweite Verbreitung der methode. 40-jährige endoprothetische Erfahrung deckt aber zwangsläufig Schwachstellen auf, mit denen sich der Verschleiß und die Lockerungsraten erklären. Prothesendesign, Materialwahl der Implantate und der Gleitpaarung, Verankerungskonzept und letztlich die Instrumentierung stehen dabei gleichwertig nebeneinander.

Das Interface Implantat/Knochen hat sich als äußerst anfällig gegenüber irritativen Reizen erwiesen. Mechanische Instabilität, Korrosions- und Abriebprodukte induzieren die Bildung von Granulationsgewebe. Durch Osteoklastenstimulierung kommt es zur Knochenresorption, schließlich lockert sich das Implantat. Der Abbauprozeß führt zu großen Defekthöhlen, die schwer angehbar sind.

Für uns hatte die Suche nach sicheren „zementfreien" Lösungen schon lange Zeit Vorrang, obwohl auch wir mit Verbesserung der Zementzusammensetzung der Zementiertechnik die Ergebnisse herkömmlicher Endoprothetik zu optimieren versuchten. In unser Bild paßten die skandinavischen Mitteilungen von PE-induzierten Prothesenlockerungen und wir waren deshalb erstaunt, von Older aus Guildford zu hören, der bei der Kaplan-Meier-Analyse eine 25-Jahres Überlebensrate von 85% herkömmlich operierter Charnley-Prothesen fand. Hier ist nicht die Zeit, detailliert über Grundsätzliches zu diskutieren.

Nur soviel: Beim Prothesendesign fordern wir formschlüssige Implantatlager, glauben aber auf eine „anatomische Form" wegen des Knochenremodelling verzichten zu können. Die Implantation hat am physiologischen Ort der Lasteinleitung zu erfolgen, also in der Kortikalis der Pfanneneingangsebene des Acetabulum und proximal am Femur. Dabei soll nur wenig tragfähiges Knochenmaterial aufgeopfert werden.

Primärstabilität ist Voraussetzung für Osseointegration. Aber Stabilität allein sichert noch kein gutes Langzeitresultat. Weller führt dabei die Knochenbiologie in's Feld, denn der Knochen als lebendes Gewebe reagiert auf Wechselbelastungen mit einem ständigen Remodelling. Distal durch Pressfit verankerte Schäfte neigen infolge pendelartigem Dauerschwingen häufig zu proximaler Auslockerung mit der Symptomatik des Oberschenkelschaftschmerzes. Daß wir mit der konsequenten proximalen Verankerung richtig liegen, zeigen das Ausbleiben dieser Beeinträchtigung ebenso wie die Röntgenverläufe. Bei der zementfreien Verankerung hat sich – nicht nur bei uns – sowohl an der Pfanne wie am Schaft Titan bewährt. Dabei wird als Ursache für die Stimulation des „bone on growth" durch Titanlegierungen eine Reaktion zwischen der Titanoxydoberfläche und dem organischen aminosäurehaltigen Material der Umgebung diskutiert. Wir verwenden zusätzlich Hydroxylapatitbeschichtungen, nachdem einerseits seit Osborn deren Effektivität gesichert und deren Anfälligkeit durch homologes Aufbringen gleichmäßig dünner Schichten unterdessen beherrscht ist. Soweit zum Design und zur Prothesenfixierung.

Nun zur Gleitpaarung:

Auf die Materialen herkömmlicher Endoprothesen sei nicht besonders eingegangen. Nach der Erkenntnis, daß Abriebpartikel, gleich welcher Art – auch inerter Materialien – immer dann die Gefahr einer Auslockerung bringen, wenn durch deren Volumen die Kapazität implantatnaher Phagozyten überschritten wird und weil Polyaethylenteilchen eine zytochemische Reaktion hervorrufen, die zu einer Osteolyse führen können, galt es Abrieb zu minimieren, besser zu vermeiden. Materialkundliche Studien müssen dabei zur Keramik führen:

Dieser Werkstoff wird in der Industrie überall dort eingesetzt, wo besondere Härte, Druckfestigkeit, optimale Gleiteigenschaften, geringer Abrieb, Thermo- und Chemostabilität benötigt werden. Für die Medizin wird der Werkstoff obendrein durch sein inertes Verhalten interessant und unter den bekannten Werkstoffen bieten die Al_2O_3-Keramiken für die Langzeitfunktionsstabilität hochbelasteter Endoprothesen beste Voraussetzungen. Das Material muß nur anatomie-, belastungs- und letztlich materialgerecht eingesetzt werden. Biokeramiken sind der einzige langjährig in situ bewährte Werkstoff, der der Natur hinsichtlich Gleitverhalten und Verschleiß am nächsten kommt. Die Keramiken unterliegen keiner chemischen Veränderung. Da kein Material eines theoretisch möglichen Verschleißes in Lösung geht, hat das Immunsystem auch keine Möglichkeit, den Fremdkörper zu erkennen. Die Acanzerogenität ist erwiesen. Durch die stabile bipolare Sauerstoffanordnung an der Al_2O_3-Oberfläche kommt es zur Bindung wässriger Umgebungsflüssigkeiten, damit zu einer filmartigen Benetzung mit eiweißhaltigen Lösungen, die nicht nur als eigentlich nicht benötigte Selbstschmierung, vor allem als Maskierung gegenüber Abstoßreaktionen wirkt. Vergleichbare Eigenschaften gehen anderen Materialkombinationen nachweislich ab. Insbesondere bei Metall/Metallpaarungen muß mit schädlicher Ionenabgabe, mit fretting, in jedem Fall mit höherem Verschleiß gerechnet werden. Die mechanischen Eigenschaften der Biokeramiken, insbesondere der Al_2O_3-Keramik, wurden in den vergangenen 10 Jahren wesentlich verbessert. Die Ergebnisse der heutigen Keramikgeneration lassen sich nicht mit denen vor 1983 erhobenen vergleichen. Werkstoffschäden bei Keramiken heutiger Güte sind nur dann möglich, wenn z. B. spannungsphysikalische Regeln mißachtet werden, deutlicher, wenn mit diesem Werkstoff nicht materialgerecht umgegangen wird. Es entfallen in jedem Fall einschränkende Kriterien wie Stoßempfindlichkeit und die Forderung nach höchst exakter Positionierung der Implantate, um Verschleiß zu vermeiden. Aus der nach wie begrenzten Biegefestigkeit ergibt sich an statisch belasteten Gelenken die Notwendigkeit, Metallkeramikverbundimplantate zu verwenden. So werden materialseitige Überforderungen vermieden.

Nach der Analyse der Schadensfälle sahen wir keine Notwendigkeit für materialseitige Änderungen. In die Überprüfung einbezogen sind 10-Jahres-Ergebnisse des alten Stufenschaftes und auch die Ergebnisse mit der monolithischen Keramikschraubpfanne, mit der wir 7% Lockerungen aufdeckten. Damit liegt die Schadensrate zwar immer noch im Rahmen der von der konventionellen Endoprothetik her bekannten. Sie erschien aber reduzierbar, da die Analyse der Schaftlockerungen punktuelle Verklemmungen an der proximal lateralen und distal medialen 5 mm erhabenen Stufe erkennen ließ. Die punktuelle Abstützung führte zu Kippinstabilitäten. Die Gefahr der Abkippung wird jetzt mit einer Stufenverkleinerung vermieden, die obendrein eine bessere Anpassung an die anatomischen Gegebenheiten bei weiterhin gewährleisteter proximaler Lasteinleitung bringt. Das dem inneren Femurausguß angenäherte Schaftdesign unterstützt die großflächige Lastverteilung und wirkt partiellen Relativbewegungen entgegen. Zudem bringt der oväläre Querschnitt die notwendige Rotationsstabilität. Die Analyse der 7% klinisch überwiegend stummen Pfannenkippungen (Buschatzky 1992) zeigte stets eine Kippung mit leichter Rotationskomponente im Sinne einer Abflachung der Pfanneneingangsebene. Die Klärung bleibt hypothetisch:

Wir nehmen an, daß in diesen Fällen die nicht einfache Fixierung des Gewindes nur teilweise oder gar nicht kortikal erfolgte. Die keramikmaterialbedingte, grobe Gestalt des Gewindes ist mögliche Ursache. Wir gingen auf einen Titangewindering mit peripher liegendem feinen selbstschneidenden Gewinde über, der zur Fixierung eines Keramikinserts analog zum Schaft einen selbsthemmenden Innenkonus erhielt. Und da zahlreiche Publikationen belegen, daß bei konischer Gestaltung der Pfanne höhere Druckkräfte besser in den Knochen eingeleitet werden können, damit gleichzeitig eine zusätzliche Kippsicherung gewährleistet ist, hat die aktuelle Pfanne einen konischen Querschnitt.

Eine schnelle ossäre Integration erwarten wir von der Hydroxylapatitbeschichtung an Pfanne und proximalem Schaft. Immer wieder auf die mögliche Gefahr des Abplatzens angesprochen, können wir nur auf die bisherigen problemlosen klinischen und röntgenologischen Verläufe verweisen.

Um unterschiedlichen Ausgangssituationen ebenso wie der Forderung nach reduzierter Lagerhaltung und wirtschaftliche Implantatherstellung Rechnung zu tragen wurde das Design der zementfreien Version dem der zementierten angeglichen. Für beide wird das gleiche Instrumentarium verwendet. Beide Schäfte erhielten den 12-/14er Eurokonus zur Koppelung mit 32 mm und 28 mm Keramik- oder Metallköpfen. Damit erschließen sich mit dem Modulsystem folgende Kombinationsmöglichkeiten der Gleitpartner:

Keramik/Keramik, Keramik/Polyaethylen und Metall/Polyaethylen. Diesem neuen System liegen unsere mehr als 25-jährigen Erfahrungen mit zementfreien Implantaten und Aluminiumoxydkeramik/Keramikgleitpartnern zugrunde. Da bei den Implantatanteilen stets auf Funktionstrennung geachtet wurde, werden den Werkstoffen und den Prothesenkomponenten nur ihre optimalen Eigenschaften abverlangt. Das ist wohl der wesentliche Grund für die Funktionssicherheit, die die klinischen Ergebnisse widerspiegeln:

Für zementfreie Implantate sind die ersten 2 auf die Implantation folgenden Jahre ohne Frage besonders wichtig. Die Ergebnisse fallen auch für uns mit 90% „sehr gut" und „gut" bewerteten Operationen unerwartet positiv aus, zumal 3 Mißerfolge auf fehlerhafte Operationstechnik zurückgehen und die 2 aufgetretenen Keramikmaterialversager ihre Ursache in Spannungsspitzen am Rand des ursprünglich verwendeten Keramikinserts der Pfanne haben. Das führte dann zur jetzigen Form, bei der das Insert total vom Titanschraubring gefaßt ist. Die operationstechnischen Fehler betrafen den Schaft. Bei der knöchernen Präparation muß unbedingt auf den Erhalt des proximalen Implantlagers geachtet werden, dem die ursprüngliche Operationsanleitung nicht Rechnung trug. Ein Operationsteam favorisierte den „südlichen Zugang". Daß dieser gegenüber den ansonsten zur Anwendung kommenden transglutäalen ungünstiger ist, beweisen dabei beobachtete ungünstigere Implantatpositionierungen sowie Luxationstendenzen, die ansonsten nicht beobachtet wurden. Als völlig problemlos erwies sich die Pfanne, bei der sowohl die richtige Auswahl der Größe als auch die Positionierung und ihre stabile Verankerung durch deren gute Ergebnisse bestätigt werden. Die röntgenologisch nachweisbare sichere Osteointegration von Pfanne und Schaft ohne bindegewebige Zwischenschicht in über 98% sprechen für das Prothesendesign, aber auch für die Hydroxylapatitbeschichtung. Bemerkenswert ist der Erfolg von prophylaktischen Maßnahmen, die den Infektionen, Embolien und paraarticulären Ossifikationen galten. Letztlich trägt auch das Ausbleiben des von früheren Implantaten her gewohnten mehrmonatigen Oberschenkelschmerzes zum positiven Gesamtergebnis bei. Mehrfache Veränderungen beim Werkzeug sichern unterdessen die einfache und wenig kraftfordernde Handhabung. Es bleiben beim Axissystem nur wenige Punkte, die einer weiteren Verbesserung bedürfen. Vordringlich ist nach wie vor eine praktikablere Handhabung des Keramikinserts und das Arbeiten an weiterer Optimierung der Keramikmaterialkenndaten, um das unterdessen an der Hüfte Erreichte auf andere statisch belastete Gelenke, insbesondere das Knie, übertragen zu können.

Zusammenfassung

Bei der weltweiten Verbreitung herkömmlicher prothetischer Methoden, einer unterdessen in die Millionen gehenden Patientenzahl, allein in Deutschland jährlich mehr als 120.000 operierten Coxarthrosen, hat sich ein konstanter Anteil von Mißerfolgen eingestellt. Die mittlere Haltbarkeit der herkömmlichen Endoprothesenmaterialen und der Verankerungszemente liegt bei 12–15 Jahren. Das wird zum Problem, weil die Zahl derer steigt, die aufgrund ihrer Lebenserwartung haltbarere als die bisher verwendeten Endoprothesen benötigen. Hinzu kommen Berichte über vorzeitige Polyaethylen-, PMMA- und Titan bedingte Endopothesenlockerungen. Unterdessen ist das Konzept der zementfreien Endoprothesenverankerung etabliert. Totales Pressfit einerseits und proximale Lasteinleitung am Schaft bzw. Kortikalis in der Eingangsebene der Pfanne anderseits stehen in Konkurrenz. Weniger einheitlich wurde die Frage der Endoprothesengrundmaterialien und der Gleitpaarungen angegangen. In unserer Klinik wird seit 1974 die Al_2O_3Keramik/Keramikhartgleitpaarung favorisiert. Die Überprüfung der klinischen Verläufe bestätigt die grundsätzliche Eignung des Materials und des zum Einsatz gekommenen Prothesendesigns. So war Materialversagen auch bei der zunächst verwendeten Frialit-Keramik bei uns nie ein Problem und die Erfolgsrate der bis 1993 verwendeten Endoprothesen mit „altem Stufenschaft" und „monolithischer Keramikpfanne" war mit 7% „schlecht" im Ergebnis durchaus der herkömmlichen Endoprothesen im Rahmen deren Gesamthaltbarkeit ebenbürtig.

Im Referat wird das aktuelle Endoprothesenkonzept des „Axis-Systems" vorgestellt, das die Schwachstellen der vorangegangenen Generationen umgeht:

Statt der monolithischen Keramikpfanne eine neu entwickelte hydroxylapatitbeschichtete konische Metallpfanne mit selbstschneidendem, peripherwärtigem Schraubgewinde und einem selbsthemmenden „Innenkonus", der ein Al_2O_3-Keramikinsert fixiert. Der ebenfalls hydroxylapatitbeschichtete Titanschaft verwendet die ursprünglich aus unserer Klinik kommende, unterdessen zum Standard gewordene proximale Lasteinleitung sowie modifizierte Stufen, die sich besser der anatomischen Vorgabe anpassen und die lastaufnehmende Oberfläche um mehr als 50% vergrößert. Im Hinblick auf das knöcherne Remodelling wird auf die bei anderen Systemen teilweise favorisierte anatomische Form mit „Rechts-/Links-Version" verzichtet. Mit einem vorwiegend motorgetriebenen Instrumentarium gestaltet sich das Implantieren wenig zeitaufwendig, sicher, wobei der transgluteäale Zugang favorisiert wird. Die bisherigen klinischen Ergebnisse scheinen das Konzept zu bestätigen. Als völlig problemlos erweist sich die Pfanne. Die 3% Fehlverläufe am Schaft sind auf Implantationsfehler zurückzuführen, was dem System nicht angelastet werden kann. Eine neue Operationsanweisung trägt dem Rechnung. Keramik-Materialversagen trat in 2 Fällen in Form von Randausbrüchen am ursprünglich nicht vom Metall umgebenen Pfanneninsert auf. Ursache sind wahrscheinliche Spannungsspitzen, dem das neue Design Rechnung trägt. Patientenseitig werden die Endoprothesen von Anfang an problemlos toleriert, zumal kein Fremdkörpergefühl oder Oberschenkelschmerz auftritt, was früher die Endoprothesenakzeptanz verringerte. Die Röntgenverlaufsserien bestätigen den „reaktionslosen" knöchernen Einbau sowohl an der Pfanne als auch am Schaft. Die prophylaktischen Maßnahmen, die den Infektionen, Embolien und paraarticulären Ossifikationen gelten, tragen in gleichem Umfang wie die technischen Voraussetzungen der Reinraumop's zum Gesamterfolg bei. Jetzt sind wir in Arbeiten eingebunden, die vom BMBF gefördert werden und dem Ziel gelten, das an der Hüfte Erreichte auf das Knie zu übertragen. Hier versprechen neue, von der CeramTec genutzte Verfahren eine Lösung, die durch verbesserte Materialkenndaten Formkörper zulassen, die den Gegebenheiten am Knie genügen.

1.8 The Rationale, Short-term Outcome and Early Complications of a Ceramic Couple in Total Hip Arthroplasty

N.R. Bergman, D.A. Young

Introduction

The association between high volumetric wear, polyethylene particulate debris, osteolysis and loosening in total hip arthroplasty is increasingly recognised and understood [1, 2]. This has resulted in an interest in alternative bearing couples, particularly in patients with a life expectancy of more than twenty years. Alumina ceramic bearings have been used since 1972 by Boutin [3] and 1976 by Sedel [4]. The Autophor prosthesis was used extensively in Europe and Australasia. Problems experienced included fracture of the ceramic head and accelerated wear when impingement of ceramic-on-ceramic occurred, or the ceramic was edge loaded due to vertical cup placement [5, 6]. In addition, poor osseointegration of ceramic-bone interfaces, and a high rate of loosening of cemented ceramic cups has been observed [7]. Those implants that functioned well showed the predicted low wear rate and membranes which appeared fairly inert [7]. There have been, however, several reports of osteolysis associated with large volumes of alumina ceramic wear debris generation and particles similar in size to those found in polyethylene wear debris [8,9].

The introduction of BIOLOX Forte and its use with a contemporary uncemented hip prosthesis is anticipated to avoid the problems of earlier designs. The aim of this study is to evaluate the safety of an alumina on alumina bearing surface in a cementless application by studying the instances of failure and complications and, secondly, to evaluate the efficacy of the bearing surface clinically and radiologically.

Materials and Methods

In all cases the Secur-Fit HA PSL ceramic on ceramic acetabular shell (Osteonics) was utilised. This titanium cup has rim press fit and line to line dome fit. It has an arc deposited titanium textured surface plasma sprayed with a 50 micron coating of hydroxyapatite. Additional fixation is possible with 6.5 mm dome screws. The shell rim is extended and rounded to allow recessing of the ceramic insert, avoiding any impingement contact with ceramic. The ceramic insert is BIOLOX Forte with a taper press fit inside the shell. We inserted the ceramic using a digital technique, or a suction cup holder. Internal diameters are 28 mm for cups less than 52 mm, and 32 mm for 52 mm and greater. A cup position of no more than 45° abduction and 30° or more flexion was aimed for.

The femoral component was either a Secur-Fit Plus HA femoral stem, a Secur-Fit HA stem, or an Omniflex HA stem from Osteonics (fig. 1). Each

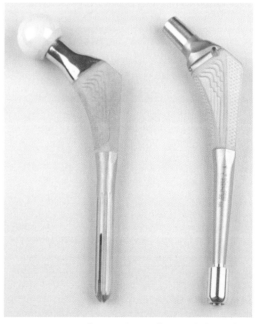

Fig. 1 Secur-Fit Plus HA femoral stem (left) and an Omniflex HA femoral stem.

has the same proximal proportional sizing and 50 micron thick hydroxyapatite coating. Distally they are designed for decreased stiffness to encourage proximal load transfer, either by fluting and a tri slot (Secur-Fit Plus HA) or a tapered stem design. They have a common instrumentation and insertion technique. Each has a C-taper 1214 trunion design. 28 mm or 32 mm BIOLOX Forte heads were used.

Patients with non inflammatory arthritis, judged to be „high demand" and with a life expectancy exceeding twenty years were entered consecutively and data collected prospectively. Inclusion and exclusion criteria are shown in Table 1.

Table 1 Inclusion Criteria

informed consent
21–75 years
not morbidly obese
usual criteria for hip arthroplasty based on history
    and examination
non inflammatory arthritis
no active infection, neurologic disorder, previous THA
    or fusion
attends for follow-up and compliant

Data has been collected pre-operatively, operatively and post-operatively using patient and surgeon completed questionnaires. Data storage and processing was using the Orthowave Outcome software and Statwave package. Post-operatively data was collected at three months, six months, one year and two years. Annual data collection is continuing.

Radiographs have been examined for implant position, fixation and stability according to Engh.

Intra-operative and post-operative problems and complications have been carefully collected. Re-operations and revisions are reported.

Results

Between October 1996 and December 1998, 139 hips in 138 patients have been implanted. Pre-operative diagnoses are shown in Table 2. Age at surgery ranged from 23 to 71 years, with a mean of 54.9 years (SD 11.1). The mean weight was 79.4kg. (46–116 kg., SD 15.0). 63% were Charnley Group A, 31% Group B and 6% Group C. All cases were primary interventions. Follow up ranges up to 24 months, but the mean for the group is 7.5 months (SD 3.8).

Table 2 Aetiology

	n	%
osteoarthritis	123	88
avascular necrosis	4	3
DDH	4	3
SUFE	2	1.5
other	6	4.5

96% utilised a postero-lateral approach and the remainder were direct lateral (trans-gluteal). Length of surgery, blood loss and length of stay were similar to the general hip replacement population (Table 3). 64% were male and 80% were discharged to home. The femoral and acetabular components utilised shown in Table 4. In 8% no screws were used in the acetabular shell. 79% had two or three screws. 82% had 32 mm femoral heads.

Table 3

male 64%	
right 53%	
length of surgery	mean 111 min (60–270)
blood loss	mean 691ml (120–2500)
length of stay	mean 8.7 days (5–21)
discharge home	80%

Table 4 Femoral Components

	n
Secur-Fit Plus HA	80
Secur-Fit HA	53
Omniflex HA	6

Pre-operatively the mean Harris hip score was 56.0 (18 to 95, SD 17.8). This increased to a mean Harris hip score of 92.8 (47 to 100, SD 10.5) at most recent follow up. The pain score improved from a mean of 14.8 to 41.0. 90% of hips were rated good or excellent (Table 5). Pre-operatively the mean Postel Merle d'Aubigne score was 10.5 (4 to 16, SD 2.5). Post-operatively this increased to 16.2 (6 to 18, SD 2.2). 83.2% were rated good or excellent (Table 6). The mean PMA pre-operative pain score was 3.5 and this increased to 5.5 post-operatively.

Table 5 Harris Hip Score at Follow-Up

Excellent	33%
Good	56.6%
Fair	7.6%
Poor	2.8%

Table 6 PMA Score at Follow-Up

Excellent	38.33%
Good	44.9%
Fair	13.1%
Poor	3.7%

Pre- and post-operative Short Form 12 (SF12) was available in 78 hips. The mean physical score improved from 31.5 pre-operatively to 46.6 at the recent review.

Radiological review is short, but the mean Engh score was 16.6 (14.0 to 19.0, SD 0.6). 100% of femoral components had either ingrowth confirmed or suspected. No hips were unstable. All acetabular components had been inserted with an abduction angle less than or equal to 45°. No cup migration or wear was detected.

Complications and re-operations are outlined in Table 7 and Table 8. The four intra-operative femoral cracks united without complication and did not affect rehabilitation. The post-operative deep vein thromboses and pulmonary embolus were treated by anticoagulation without complication. The wound seroma resolved. The heterotopic bone required no additional treatment and became asymptomatic.

Table 7

Complications (n = 19)	
intra-operative femoral crack	4
ceramic chip fracture	3
partial sciatic nerve palsy	6
wound seroma	1
DVT	2
PE	1
heterotopic ossification (Brooker2)	1
recurrent subluxation	1

Table 8

Reoperations (n = 7)	
Psoas release	1
Cup revision (subluxation)	1
Sciatic nerve exploration	4
Femoral shortening	1

The three ceramic fractures were surface flake chips off the liner. They occurred on impaction. Two were on the outer edge (fig. 2) and the third on the inner edge of the rim. The liner was changed in each case.

There were 6 partial sciatic nerve palsies. Three were associated with leg lengthening intra-operatively for hip dysplasia. One of these had an occult L5 S1 disc prolapse. One non dysplasia case was treated by acute femoral shortening. Two were in the one patient who underwent bilateral procedures, separated by six months. On one side the nerve was re-explored. Both sides resolved. One other case was acutely explored, no abnormality found and the lesion resolved.

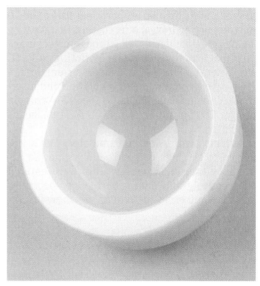

Fig. 2 Peripheral rim chip.

The case of recurrent subluxation was treated by revision of the acetabular component, providing further cup flexion and lengthening the neck by 5 mm. The psoas tendonitis failed to resolve with conservative treatment and injections. Exploration of the psoas tendon and excision of a frayed and degenerate section of the psoas tendon at the anterior rim of the cup completely resolved his pain in flexion.

There were no deep infections.

Discussion

The early clinical and radiological results in this group of ceramic-on-ceramic hip replacements are very satisfactory with Harris and PMA scores indicating early success clinically. The radiographs suggest that osseointegration is predictable, similar to that seen with CoCr-UHMPE articulations [10, 11].

Fracture of the rim of the ceramic liner was seen in three hips (2.2%). In two the chip fracture commenced on the outer edge of the lateral flat sur-

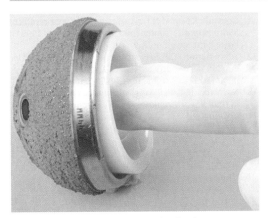

Fig. 3 Malposition resulting in edge loading on impaction.

face. A small flake was dislodged and could not be found. The fractures were difficult to see but were easy to feel. They were highlighted by blood which clung to the rough surface. The fractures represent edge loading at the rim due to malposition of the ceramic liner (fig. 3). On each occasion the liner was felt to be seated properly, to visual inspection, and was not loose when removal was attempted. Careful insertion into a dry shell with no interposing tissue is emphasised. The liner is then impacted and carefully inspected and palpated. Design changes to decrease stress on this edge and to facilitate accurate liner insertion would seem appropriate.

The third ceramic liner chip fracture occurred on the outer surface but away from the outer edge. It was due to malposition of the impactor. Flat seating of any impactor on the ceramic liner is important to avoid uneven loading or tilting at impaction.

As the chip fracture rate of the liner is about 2%, each liner should be carefully inspected after insertion. If a fracture is found, a new liner should be inserted and a search made to ensure that the fragment is not in the joint cavity.

The case of recurrent subluxation highlights the importance of cup placement. This cup was in neutral and impinged at hip flexion over 95°. The young female patient demanded hip flexion over 100° to resume her usual activities. Increasing the cup flexion and neck length resolved the problem.

A high rate of sciatic nerve injury was encountered [12, 13]. This is not bearing couple specific, but highlights the difficulties encountered in hip dysplasia with pre-operative shortening, and cases where pre existing lumbar disc prolapse is present, increasing sciatic nerve tension. Careful operative technique, protection of the sciatic nerve, measurement of leg length and offset intra-operatively and nerve tension evaluation using a straight leg raise is emphasised. We use a marker on the ischium and the greater trochanter to measure both leg length and offset. Post-operatively the limb can be nursed with some flexion at the knee, if it has been lengthened. This decreases tension on the sciatic nerve and should decrease the risk of late sciatic nerve dysfunction.

The operation for psoas tendonitis represented a pre-operative problem that did not resolve post-operatively until the psoas tendon was divided.

Summary

The early clinical and radiological results of alumina ceramic bearings in this group of young active patients is very satisfactory. Accurate surgical technique to avoid edge loading and impingement is emphasised. Chip fractures of the rim of the liner were seen in 2% of cases and may be avoided by careful insertion and possibly design changes. Attention is drawn to the sciatic nerve which is prone to injury when leg lengths are altered and in associated with co-existing lumbar disc prolapse.

References

1. Howie, D.W., et al., *The response to particulate debris* (1993). Orthop Clin North Am, **24**(4): p. 571–81.
2. Schmalzried, T.P. and P. Campbell, *Isolation and characterization of debris in membranes around total joint prostheses [letter; comment]*(1995). J Bone Joint Surg Am, **77**(10): p. 1625–6.
3. Boutin, P., et al., *The use of dense alumina-alumina ceramic combination in total hip replacement* (1988). J Biomed Mater Res, **22**(12): p. 1203–32.
4. Sedel, L., et al., *Alumina-on-alumina hip replacement. Results and survivorship in young patients*(1990). J Bone Joint Surg [Br], **72**(4): p. 658–63.
5. Kummer, F.J., S.A. Stuchin, and V.H. Frankel, *Analysis of removed autophor ceramic-on-ceramic components* (1990). J Arthroplasty, **5**(1): p. 28–33.
6. Mittelmeier, H. and J. Heisel, *Sixteen-years' experience with ceramic hip prostheses* (1992). Clin Orthop, (282): p. 64–72.
7. Nizard, R.S., et al., *Ten-year survivorship of cemented ceramic-ceramic total hip prosthesis* (1992). Clin Orthop, (282): p. 53–63.
8. Sedel, L., R. Nizard, and P. Bizot, *Massive osteolysis after ceramic on ceramic total hip arthroplasty [letter; comment]* (1998). Clin Orthop, (349): p. 273–4.

9. Yoon, T.R., et al., *Osteolysis in association with a total hip arthroplasty with ceramic bearing surfaces* (1998). J Bone Joint Surg Am, **80**(10): p. 1459-68.
10. Capello, W.N., et al., *Hydroxyapatite-coated total hip femoral components in patients less than fifty years old. Clinical and radiographic results after five to eight years of follow-up* (1997). J Bone Joint Surg Am, **79**(7): p. 1023-9.
11. Geesink, R.G. and N.H. Hoefnagels, *Six-year results of hydroxyapatite-coated total hip replacement* (1995). J Bone Joint Surg Br, **77**(4): p. 534-47.
12. Schmalzried, T.P., S. Noordin, and H.C. Amstutz, *Update on nerve palsy associated with total hip replacement* (1997). Clin Orthop, (344): p. 188-206.
13. Navarro, R.A., et al., *Surgical approach and nerve palsy in total hip arthroplasty* (1995). J Arthroplasty, **10**(1): p. 1-5.

1.9 Analysis of Wear Debris Particles from Alumina on Alumina Ceramic THA

M. Böhler, Y. Mochida, Th.W. Bauer, M. Salzer

The inflammatory reaction to small particles of wear debris appears to have influence on long term stability of total joint prostheses. Factors such as size, shape, composition of wear particles and the particle concentration in the periprosthetic tissues play a central role in the developement of aseptic loosening and osteolysis (3, 4, 6–9). Little is known about the tissue concentration and physical characteristics of wear particles originating from dense, polycrystalline Al_2O_3 ceramic used for THAs (4). Since a particle size of 1 μm is at the lower limit for light microscopy, more sensitive methods have been developed to evaluate submicron debris in tissue membranes from revised arthroplasties (2,5).

The purposes of this study was to describe the histologic findings of tissues around failed, ceramic-ceramic total hip prostheses, to quantify the approximate concentration and composition of debris particles, to determine the origin of the particles, and to compare the properties of particles from ceramic-ceramic implants with a limited group of implants identical except for the use of a modular polyethylene acetabular insert.

In the present study we compared the periprosthetic tissues of: Group 1) a series of 9 cementless monobloc alumina ceramic sockets and ball heads (Rosenthal-Technik AG, manufactured before ISO 6474) on Co-based alloy stems without (n = 6) and with bone cement fixation (n = 3) [mean implantation time 131 mos (range 11–237 mos)] (1) with Group 2) a series of 11 cementless modular Ti sockets with alumina ceramic inlays and ball heads (BIOLOX®, Cerasiv, ISO 6474) on cementless Ti-alloy stems [mean implantation time 33 mos(range 7–60 mos)]. These results will then be compared with results from Group 3) a series of 7 cases with identical prostheses as Group 2 but with modular polyethylene acetabular inserts (UMWP RCH 1000; Hoechst, Germany) [mean implantation time 42.1 months (range 18–61 mos.)]

According to a standard protocol (2,5) the specimen blocks were freed from embedding media (Paraffin or PMMA), digested in conc.nitric acid and the ceramic, metal and polyethylene wear particles counted in water-dispersant solution using a Coulter Multisizer (size range 0.5 to 10 μm) The sizes and compositions of all particles collected on filters were analysed by SEM and EDAX.

The calculated mean total number of wear particles/g /yr was $0.70 \pm 0.79 \times 10^9$ for Group 1, $1.62 \pm 2.13 \times 10^9$ for Group 2 and $4.26 \pm 6.38 \times 10^9$ for Group 3. With the number of samples available, there is a significantly higher tissue particle concentration for the ceramic-polyethylene hips (Group 3), when compared to the ceramic-ceramic hips in (Groups 1 and 2).

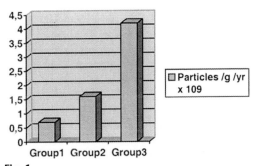

Fig. 1

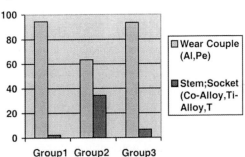

Fig. 2

Table 1 Size range and average size for each particle type determined by SEM (in μm)

Particle	Size measure	Filter	Group 1 and 2	Group 3
Al	Over all size range		0,13 – 78,38	0,18 – 63,25
	Average size	0.1 μm filter	0,41 – 0,36	0,32 – 0,12
	Average size	0.4 μm filter	1,61 – 1,83	1,51 – 0,98
TiAlV	Over all size range		0,18 – 57,75	0,26 – 34,38
	Average size	0.1 μm filter	0,45 – 0,30	0,35 – 0,09
	Average size	0.4 μm filter	1,52 – 1,52	1,37 – 0,70
Ti	Over all size range		0,22 – 52,25	0,22 – 66,00
	Average size	0.1 μm filter	0,50 – 0,24	0,42 – 0,05
	Average size	0.4 μm filter	1,23 – 0,97	3,18 – 4,90
Co	Over all size range		0,26 – 75,63	
	Average size	0.1 μm filter	0,49 – 0,33	
	Average size	0.4 μm filter	1,65 – 1,23	
UHMWPE	Over all size range		*	0,13 – 781,00
	Average size	0.1 μm filter	*	0,40 – 0,20
	Average size	0.4 μm filter	*	2,36 – 2,10

* Not Applicable

The composition of particles in the periprosthetic tissues showed mainly ceramic particles in Group 1, 2/3 Alumina particles and 1/3 metallic particles in Group 2, and mainly polyethylene particles in Group 3.

Size range and average size for each type of particles on each filter are shown in Table 3. Polyethylene particles have a larger size range than the other type of particles, but with the numbers available, no significant difference in average size could be detected among the different types of particles present (alumina, cobalt-alloy, titanium-aluminum-vanadium alloy, titanium, polyethylene). Similarly, no significant difference in average particle size could be detected between the groups of cases. Very few particles smaller than 0.2 micrometer were identified.

In our study it was possible to compare wear particles from tissues around the „old" alumina-ceramic, produced before ISO 6474, with those around the „newer" ceramic, produced according to ISO 6474 and for the first time this study compares the composition, size and concentration of particles between matched modular hip implants of nearly identical design except for the UHMWPE articulating surfaces. By applying a well documented tissue digestion and particle counting protocol it was also possible to compare our present results with the results of such a particle analysis from tissues around metal-on-poly ethylene prostheses, previously published by one of the co-authors (2, 5).

With respect to size of alumina particles we could find no significant differences between the „older" and the „newer" ceramic. But we found a relationship between implantation time and percentage of particles larger than 10 μm which may be attributed to more fatigue and abrasion of the alumina gliding surface in the „older" ceramic, a phenomenon which was not encountered in the „newer" group in this extent. The results are in contrast to the publication of Lerouge et al. (4) who reported an average alumina particle size of 0.44 ± 0.25 μm without any information on particles greater than 1.2 μm.

The unique composition of implants in this study allowed us to determine the origin of most of the wear particles. Both, acetabular component and modular head in group 1 were composed of alumina ceramic, while the femoral stem was made of Co-based alloy. The majority of particles in Group 1 were composed of alumina (94.4%), with only 2.2% CoCr-particles from the femoral stem. In Group 2, the ceramic insert and modular head was alumina ceramic, the acetabular backing was c.p. titanium, and the femoral stem was Ti- alloy. Only 63.6% of the particles in Group 2 were alumina, with 29.9% Ti-alloy from the femoral stem and 4.5% pure Ti from the metal backing which is in contrast to an earlier study of Hirakawa et al. (2) where the authors speculated that most of the metal particles were from the socket prostheses. In Group 3 an identical prosthesis was used as in Group 2 but with a UHMW polyethylene insert as the only difference. The composition of particles was mainly polyethyle (80%) few Al particles (13,5%) and some metallic debris (6,5%).

With respect to the overall particle concentration (particles/gram tissue) we could not identify any significant difference between Groups 1 and 2 but there was a significantly higher particlew concentration found in periprosthetic tissues of Group 3 which was due the high rate of PE-particles. Comparing our recent results with earlier published data of other wear couples, the use of ceramic-ceramic bearings resulted in a 2–22 times lower particle concentation in the periprosthetic tissues (2, 5).

Controlled, prospective studies are required to definitively demonstrate reduced wear debris accumulation in ceramic-on-ceramic hip arthroplasty, but our results suggest a relatively low rate of particle accumulation in tissues adjacent to failed ceramic-on-ceramic implants, when compared to alumina-on-polyethylene articulations of an identical design. Nevertheless, careful operative technique with correct positioning of the implanted prostheses is necessary to avoid excessive ceramic wear production and care must be taken to avoid impingement between the femoral neck and the rim of the implant, a situation previously associated with osteolysis in one case 10. Based on the present results and our clinical experience we continue to recommend alumina ceramic as a gliding couple in total hip arthroplasty.

References

1. Böhler M, Knahr K, Plenk jr H, Walter A, Salzer M, Schreiber V, Long-Term Results of Uncemented Alumina Acetabular Implants. *J.Bone Joint Surg. [Br]* 1994, 76B, 53–59
2. Hirakawa K, Bauer TW, Stulberg BN, Wilde AH, Secic M: Characterization and Comparison of Wear Debris from Failed Total Hip Implants of Different Sites *J.Bone Joint Surg. [Am]* 1996, 78A, 1235–1243
3. Howie DW., Tissue Response in Relation to Type of wear aprticles Around Failed Hip Arthroplasties. *Journ. Arthroplasty.* 1990, Vol 5. No. 4, 337–348
4. Lerouge S, Huk O, Yahia LH, Sedel L., Characterization of in vivo wear debris from ceramic-ceramic total hip arthroplasties .*Journ of Biomedical Materials Research,* 1996, Vol 32, 627–633
5. Margevicius KJ, Bauer TW, McMahon JT, Brown SA, Eng D, Merritt K., Isolation and Characterization of Debris in Membranes around Total Joint Prostheses., *J. Bone Joint Surg. [Am]* 1994, 76A, 1664–1675,
6. Merritt K.. Role of medical materials, both in implant and surface applications, in immune response and in resistance to infections. *Biomaterials* 1984, 5: 47–
7. Plenk H.jr., Biocompatibility of Ceramics in Joint Prostheses. In: D.F. Williams, ed., *Biocompatibility of Orthopedic Implants.* Vol. I., CRC-Press Inc., Boca Raton, FL, 1982, 269–295
8. Salzer M, Knahr K, Plenk HJr, Long Term Clinical and Histological Evaluation Of Bioceramic Total Hip Endoprostheses. *Orthopaedics,* 1981, Vol 4/No 11, 1231–
9. Sedel et al.: Prostaglandin E2 Level in tissue surrounding aseptic failed total hips. Effects of materials. *Arch.Orthop. Trauma. Surg.,* 1992, 111(5), 255–8,
10. Wirganowicz PZ, Thomas BJ: Massive Osteolysis after Ceramic on Ceramic Total Hip Arthroplasty. *Clin. Orthop.* 1997, No 338, 100–104

2 Reliability – Clinical Aspects

2.1 Ceramic Ball Head Retrieval Data

G. Willmann

Since the 1970's when first it was realized that the properties of alumina ceramics could be exploited to provide better implants for orthopedic applications, the field has expanded enormously. Applications depend on the fact that alumina ceramics are corrosion resistant, offer an excellent biocompatibility, are synoviaphil, are extremely hard and scratch resistant, and provide wear characteristics suitable for bearing surfaces in total hip replacement (1). Resultant orthopedic use has enjoyed more than 20 years' clinical success. Up to the present more than 2.5 million alumina femoral heads have been implanted. Their popularity is based on two facts: extremely low wear rate and reliability.

It is a fact that materials scientists have substantially improved the properties of wear resistant alumina, e. g. mechanical strength which is correlated to reliability, i.e. fracture in vivo. There are three generation of medical-grade alumina. The latest one is an alumina that is **h**ot **i**sostatic **p**ressed (HIP), laser marked and proof-tested (2, 3). Some important properties are listed in table 1.

Table 1 Some characteristics of BIOLOX®forte ceramics (Typical values)

Property	1st generation	2nd generation	3rd generation
Bending strength (MPa)	> 450	> 500	> 550
Density (g /cm^3)	3.94	3.96	3.98
Grain size (µm)	≤ 4.5	≤ 3.2	≤ 1.8
HIP	no	no	yes
Laser Marking	no	no	yes
100% control	yes	yes	yes
Proof-test	no	no	yes

In 1995 Toni (4) published a review reporting a list of fracture rates which ranged between 0% for today's ceramics and up more than 10% for ceramics manufactured before 1980. It is important to note that these high fracture rates were caused by materials manufactured by companies that are not on the market anymore. These old aluminas had a low density, a very coarse microstructures, and are not in compliance with specifications valid today, e.g. ISO 6474 and ASTM F 603. The in vivo fracture rates of the most commonly used ceramic BIOLOX®forte have been analyzed by various groups, e.g. Semlitsch of Sulzer medica published reports based on more than half a million heads (5, 6). CeramTec's reports are based on more than 1.5 million heads (7-9). The fracture rate of ceramic femoral BIOLOX®forte heads are listed in table 2.

Table 2 Fracture rate of BIOLOX® forte ceramics

1st generation	2nd generation	3rd generation
0.026%	0.014%	0.004%
26 : 100,000	14 : 100,000	4 : 100,000

Analyzing the clinical experience of 25 years it can be concluded that the technical improvements are offering reliability (3, 4-6, 8, 9).

Results of wear tests with a hip simulator and investigations of retrievals prove that the wear rate of the wear couple BIOLOX®forte-on-BIOLOX®forte is extremely low (10-12).

References

1. Clarke I, Willmann G (1994) Structural Ceramics in Orthopedics. In: Cameron HU (ed) Bone Implant Interface. Mosby, St. Louis, Baltimore, Boston, 203-25
2. Willmann G, Pfaff HG, Richter H (1995) Enhanced Safety of Ceramic femoral Hedas for Use with Hip Joint Endoprotheses (Steigerung der Sicherheit von keramischen Kugelköpfen für Hüftendoprothesen) Biomed Technik 40: 342-346
3. Heros R, Willmann G (1998) Ceramics in Total Hip Arthroplasty: History, Mechanical Properties, Clinical results and Current Manufacturing State of the Art. Sem Arthroplasty 9: 114-122
4. Toni A et al (1995) Ceramics in Total Hip Arthroplasty. In: Wise DL (eds) Encyclopedic Hand-

book of Biomaterials and Bioengineering. Marcel Dekker, Inc New York, Basel, Hong Kong 1501–1544

5 Semlitsch M, Dawihl W (1994) Basic Requirements of Alumina Ceramic in Artificial hip Joint Balls in Articulation with Polyethylen Cups. In: Buchhorn GH, Willert HG (eds.): Technical Principles, Design and Safety of Joint Implants. Hogrefe & Huber Publ Seattle, Toronto, Bern, Göttingen 99–101

6 Semlitsch M, Weber H, Steger R (1995) Biomed Technik 40: 347–355

7 Willmann G (1998) Ceramics for Total Hip Replacement – What a Surgeon Should Know. Orthopaedics 21: 173–177

8 Willmann G (1996) How Safe are Ceramic Femoral Heads for Total Hip Arthroplasty? (Wie sicher sind keramische Kugelköpfe für Hüftendoprothesen?) Mat wiss u Werkstofftechnik 27: 280–286

9 Willmann G (1998) Survival Rate and Reliability of Ceramic Femoral Heads for Total Hip Arthroplasty. (Überlebenswahrscheinlichkeit und Sicherheit von keramischen Kugelköpfen für Hüftendoprothesen.) Mat u Werkstofftechnik 29: 595–604

10 Henßge EJ, Bos I, Willmann G (1994) Al_2O_3 against Al_2O_3 combination in hip endoprotheses – Histologic investigations with semiquantitave grading of revision and autopsy cases and abrasion measures. J Materials Science Mat in Medicine 5: 657–661

11 Refior HJ, Plitz W, Walter W (1997) Ex vivo and in vivo analysis og the alumina/alumina bearing system for hip joint prostheses. In: Sedel L, Rey Ch (eds) Bioceramics 10, Pergamon, Elsevier Sci Ltd, Oxford, 127–130

12 Taylor SK, Serekian P, Manley M (1998) Wear Performance of a Contemporary Alumina – alumina Bearing Couple Under Hip Joint Simulation. 44th Ann meeting Orthop Res Soc, March 15–19 1998 New Orleans, Louisiana 51–9

2.2 CeramTec's Recommendations for Revision when Using BIOLOX®forte Femoral Heads

G. Willmann

Abstract

CeramTec's advice is not to mount a ceramic femoral head on prior (damaged) tapers at revision. For details see CeramTec's OP-Chart.

Revision surgery in THR

Revision surgery are performed due to various reasons. An excellent review about the statistics on revisions and a list of typical reasons for revisions can be found in the Swedish register on THR revisions (1).

Quite often the acetabular component has to be revised while the stem stays in situ because it is well fixed. In cases like that it is common practice that the femoral heads is taken off to gain more space for performing the revision of the acetabular component. When taking off the femoral head there is a chance that the metal taper of the stem is damaged.

Potential for damaging the metal taper at revision

Today's high reliability of ceramic heads (2, 3, 4) is based on the precision of the metal taper cone on the femoral stem side. The surface of the metal taper is particularly vulnerable during surgery. If the surface of the metal taper is damaged the risk of fracture is enhanced. Willmann (5), Heimke (6), Clarke and Willmann (7) have reviewed the specifications of today's metal tapers and the problems that may arise when the metal taper is not according to specifications or is damaged due to mishandling. We have investigated the burst strength of ceramic femoral heads in our laboratory using the procedures according to the international standard ISO 7206-5 (8) and FDA guidance document (9). The test results prove that the burst strength of a ceramic head has been reduced when the head was mounted on a damaged metal taper, e.g. when the taper was scratched with an instrument or the taper is easily damaged when taking off a femoral head during revision surgery.

CeramTec's advice

Therefore CeramTec's advice is not to mount a ceramic femoral head on prior (damaged) tapers at revision. For details see appendix I.

Future activities

In session 2 of the 4th International CeramTec Symposium 1999 this topic was discussed focussing on how to take off the femoral head and how to replace it. Four speakers had agreed to give short presentations what procedure would be the best. These four statements are published in this chapter. Speakers from the floor gave statements, too.

On the Symposium there was no consensus on this important topic. Therefore it was decided to go on with the discussion, to compile more experimental results and to report on the 5th Int. CeramTec Symposium in 2000. May be a consensus can be found then.

2.2 CeramTec's Recommendation for Revision when Using BIOLOX®forte Femoral Heads

BIOLOX® forte – Surgical Instructions Card

BIOLOX® forte components can be resterilized as often as required!

Damage Prevention

Sterilization: After sterilization in the autoclave BIOLOX® forte components should not be subject to sudden cooling, for instance by immersion in water. Always allow BIOLOX® forte components to cool down slowly.

Taper-fit connection

Care should be taken to ensure the perfect fit of the BIOLOX® forte component on the taper of the stem. Only use 12/14 BIOLOX® forte components in conjunction with 12/14 stem tapers. The same applies to tapers sized 14/16.

BIOLOX® forte components should be used exclusively on prosthetic stems which have been approved by CeramTec.

Fixation of the BIOLOX® forte component on the prosthetic stem

Objective: perfect fit of the BIOLOX® forte component on the stem taper.

The plastic cap which protects the taper against damage should be removed only immediately prior to fitting the trial head.

Before fitting the BIOLOX® forte component on the stem:

- Ensure the stem taper has been thoroughly rinsed with water.
- Ensure the stem taper is dry by using a clean swab.
- Ensure the stem taper and the taper of the femoral head has been thoroughly inspected.
- Ensure any foreign bodies such as tissue residues and bone or cement particles have been removed from both tapers.

To fit the BIOLOX® forte component on the stem taper, exert slight axial pressure on the femoral head and twist it simultaneously until the femoral head sits firmly on the stem and can no longer be moved.

Place the nylon femoral head impactor on the pole of the BIOLOX® forte femoral head and tap home with a mallet in an axial direction so as to firmly jam the femoral head on the stem taper.

Hotline: +49 – 7153 – 6 11-314

BIOLOX® forte – Surgical Instructions Card

Attention:
Never hit a BIOLOX® forte femoral head with a metal hammer.

Replacement of femoral heads
BIOLOX® forte femoral heads should always be replaced by a metal femoral head.
Never reuse a BIOLOX® forte femoral head on a different stem once the femoral head has been impacted on a stem and has then been removed. When revision of a BIOLOX® forte femoral head is required and the prosthetic stem remains in situ, always revise with a metal femoral head.
Never use the BIOLOX® forte femoral head on a damaged taper or on a taper which does not fit the femoral head.

Reoperation in case of fracture of the ceramic femoral head:
Make sure the ceramic femoral head is replaced by a metal femoral head. Replace the polyethylene cup. It will probably be necessary to replace the prosthetic stem.

- Make sure all ceramic particles have been removed.
- Replace the PE cup – even if it seems to be in good condition and well fixed.

The above instructions must be complied to in order to ensure the successful use of BIOLOX® forte.

Please do not autoclave this Instruction Card.

CeramTec AG
Innovative Ceramic Engineering
Medical Products Division
Fabrikstraße 23–29
D-73207 Plochingen
Phone +49–7153–611-522
Fax +49–7153–611-496

CeramTec
THE CERAMIC EXPERTS

Hotline: +49 – 7153 – 611-314

References

1. Malchau H, Herberts P (1996) Prognosis of Total Hip Replacement; Revision and Re-Revision Rate in THR: A Revision – Risk Study of 148.359 Primary Operations. SCI Exhibition 53rd AAOS, Atlanta Feb 22–26, 1996
2. Heros R, Willmann G (1998) Ceramics in Total Hip Arthroplasty: History, Mechanical Properties, Clinical results and Current Manufacturing State of the Art. Seminars of Arthroplasty 9: 114–122
3. Toni A, Sudanese A, Busanelli L, Zappoli FA, Brizo L, Giunti A (1998) Cementless arthroplasty using alumina ceramics as a coating and bearing material In: Sedel L, Cabanela ME(eds) Hip Surgery – Materials and Developments. Martin Dunitz, London, 267–276
4. Lerouge S., L'Hocine Yahia, Sedel L (1998) Alumina ceramics for the femoral head of a hip prostheses In: Sedel L, Cabanela ME (eds) Hip Surgery – Materials and Developments. Martin Dunitz, London, 31–40
5. Willmann, G (1993) Das Prinzip der Konus-Steckverbindung für keramische Kugelköpfe bei Hüftgelenkprothesen. Mat-wiss u Werkstofftechnik 24: 315–319
6. Heimke, G (1993) Safety Aspects of the Fixation of Ceramic Balls on Metal Stems. Bioceramics 6: 283–288
7. Clarke, I., G. Willmann (1994) Structural Ceramics in Orthopedics In:
Cameron HU (ed) Bone Implant Interface. Mosby, St. Louis, Baltimore, Boston, Chicago, London, 203–252
8. ISO 7206-5 Implants for Surgery – Partial and Total Hip Joint Prostheses Part 5: Determination of the resistance to static load of head and neck region of stemmed femoral components. Int Standard Organization 1st ed. 1992-03-15
9. Food and Drug Administration (FDA) (1995) Guidance Document for the Preparation of Premarket Notification for Ceramic Ball Hip Systems. FDA, Washington D.C. USA 2nd ed. 1995

2.3 Vorgangsweise und Erfahrungen für den Wechsel keramischer Kugelköpfe

K. Zweymüller

Unsere Erfahrungen mit keramischen Kugelköpfen reichen auf die Mitte der 70er Jahre zurück (1). In großer Fallzahl und später fast ausschließlich wurde die Keramikkugel ab Ende des Jahres 1979 verwendet. Es fiel dies mit der Einführung des zementfreien konischen Geradschaftsystems aus geschmiedeter Titanlegierung zusammen. Die Keramikkugel artikulierte mit Polyäthylen. Anfangs waren noch zementierte Polyäthylenpfannen die überwiegend verwendeten Artikulationspartner. Ab 1981 jedoch und bis Ende 1984 wurden fast ausschließlich zementfreie Polyäthylenschraubpfannen in direkter Verankerung zum Knochen eingebaut (2, 3). Dies entsprach dem damaligen Stand des Wissens und kam dem Wunsch nach „Isoelastizität" des Implantates im Verbund mit dem Beckenknochen entgegen. Die Mißerfolge mit diesem Pfannensystem lagen im progressiven Abrieb der Pfannenaußenwand im Kontakt mit dem Knochen. Die Destruktion des Polyäthylens führte zur Ausbildung von Fremdkörpergranulationsgewebe, welches das knöcherne Pfannenlager sowie sekundär auch das Schaftlager zerstörte und zur Lockerung der Implantate führte. Mit Einführung der metal-back Pfannenschale aus Reintitan Anfang 1985 war das Problem des Polyäthylen-Granuloms weitestgehend gelöst (4). Zurück blieb jedoch eine große Zahl durchzuführender Revisionen. Diese betrafen vorwiegend die Pfannen; im Bereich der Schäfte waren Austauschoperationen signifikant seltener.

Die an uns gerichtete Herausforderung lag in der Austauschoperation bei zu belassendem Schaftimplantat. Dabei wurden wir in vielen Fällen vor das Problem des optimalen Zuganges gestellt, wobei die am Metallkonus belassene Keramikkugel ein Zugangshindernis darstellte. Sie wurde deshalb in vielen Fällen vom Konus abgeschlagen. Der Konus wurde während der Austauschoperation nach Möglichkeit vor Beschädigungen geschützt und am Schluß der Operation wurde wiederum eine Keramikkugel aufgesetzt.

In jenen Fällen, in denen die Kugel kein Zugangshindernis darstellte, ergab sich in etwa jedem zweiten Fall die Notwendigkeit, eine andere – zumeist längere Halslänge – vorzusehen. Auch in diesen Fällen wurde somit die Kugel vom Konus abgeschlagen und durch eine neue Keramikkugel ersetzt. In allen Fällen war der Gleitpartner der Keramikkugeln Polyäthylen, entweder in Form einer zementierten, zumeist aber in Form der zementfrei implantierten metal-back Pfannenschale mit Polyäthyleninlay.

Zum Abziehen der keramischen Kugel wurde fast von Anfang an ein metallischer Ausschläger verwendet, mit dem auf die Basis der Kugel geschlagen wurde. Um den Konus vor Beschädigungen zu schützen, wurde eine mehrfach zusammengelegte Kompresse zwischen Metallinstrument und Keramikkugel gelegt. Das neuerliche Aufstecken einer Keramikkugel schien uns durchaus vertretbar. Nur in Fällen von massiven Beschädigungen des Konus wurden somit in Einzelfällen Metallkugeln aufgesetzt.

Im Lichte der heute geführten Diskussionen, ob es statthaft wäre, eine neue Keramikkugel auf einen potentiell beschädigten Metallkonus aufzusetzen, können unsere Erfahrungen als durchaus positiv angesehen werden. Es sind mir bis heute keine Kugelbrüche bekannt, welche aufgrund dieser Vorgangsweise aufgetreten sind. Bei einer Zahl von Revisionseingriffen von mehreren hundert ist somit auch die Zahl der gewechselten Kugeln hoch. Diese persönliche Erfahrung erhebt jedoch keinerlei Anspruch auf Vollständigkeit, da es durchaus möglich ist, daß der eine oder andere Fall eines Kugelbruches notfallsmäßig in einem anderen Krankenhaus revidiert worden sein könnte, ohne daß wir von diesem Vorfall informiert worden wären.

Wir verwenden diese Technik der Kugelentfernung bis heute und haben keine Sorge, daß eine neuerlich aufgesetzte Keramikkugel brechen könnte. Eine vorsichtige und beschädigungsfreie

Entfernung der Kugel vom Metallkonus ist dafür die Voraussetzung.

Der immer wieder geforderte Austausch der Keramikkugel gegen eine Metallkugel erscheint uns aufgrund unserer Ergebnisse als nicht indiziert. Zu bedenken ist dabei auch, daß der zu erwartende Polyäthylenabrieb zwischen Metallkugel und Pfanne signifikant höher ist als bei einer Keramik-Polyäthylenpaarung. Eine auch nur geringe Beschädigung der Metalloberfläche würde zusätzlich zu einer exponentiellen Zunahme des abgeriebenen Polyäthylen führen. Da im Gegensatz dazu Keramikkugeln durch den Kontakt mit metallischen Gegenständen nicht beschädigt werden können, ist ihre Verwendung auch aus diesem Grunde wesentlich sicherer. Untersuchungen an explantierten Keramikkugeln mit deutlichen Schwarzverfärbungen der Kugeloberfläche wiesen Auflagerungen auf, jedoch keine Defekte (5).

Literatur

1. Zweymüller K.: Knochen- und Gelenksersatz mit biokeramischen Endoprothesen. Wien: Facultas 1978
2. Endler M., Endler F.: Theoretisch-experimentelle Grundlagen und erste klinische Erfahrungen mit einer neuen zementfreien Polyäthylenschraubpfanne bei Hüftgelenkersatz. Acta Chirurgica Austriaca, Suppl. 45, 1, 1982
3. Zweymüller K.: A cementless titanium hip endoprosthesis system. Basic research and clinical results. In: The AAOS Instructional Course Lectures, V. 35, St. Louis, C.V. Mosby, 1986
4. Zweymüller K., Lintner F., Semlitsch M.: Biologic Fixation of a Press-Fit Titanium Hip Joint Endoprosthesis. Clin. Orthop. Rel. Res., No. 235, 195–206, 1988
5. Willmann G., Kemmer U., Zweymüller K.: Investigation of Retrieved Femoral Biolox Heads. Bioceramics. Vol. 7, 377–381. Hrsg.: Andersson Ö.H., Yli-Urpo A., 1994

2.4 Revisionsstrategie nach Bruch oder Verschleiß von Keramikkomponenten

P. Griss, A. Claus, G. Scheller

Die Frage, was zu tun ist, wenn eine Keramik/Keramik-Hüftendoprothese gewechselt werden muß, kann nur auf dem Boden des derzeitigen Kenntnisstandes beantwortet werden. Dieser muß zunächst kurz rekapituliert werden. An Hand der Analyse von Gewebeproben von 26 Reoperationen von Keramik/Keramik-Kombinationen haben wir zusammen mit Willert (1) feststellen müssen, daß Keramikabriebpartikel in allen Fällen nachzuweisen waren. Sie führen zwar in der Regel nur zu moderaten Gewebereaktionen, wenn alleinig vorhanden, man findet sie aber überall im Grenzflächengewebe der Verankerung von zementfreier Pfanne und an der Zement-Knochengrenze selbst bei nicht gelockerten Schäften, ja in einzelnen Fällen sogar im Knochen der Verankerung eingelagert. Selbstverständlich auch in allen Schichten der Neokapsel. Kommt auf Grund des Versagensmechanismus (z.B. Kopfbruch) noch Metallabrieb hinzu entstehen aggressive Mischgranulome. Diese Befunde legen nahe, daß auch ein noch so gründliches Debridement die Partikel nicht vollständig entfernen kann. Daß Keramikabriebpartikel auch im Gelenkraum Wirkung entfalten können lehrt ein von uns kürzlich beobachteter Fall. Er gibt auch Hinweise zur eingangs gestellten Frage.

Zum Zeitpunkt der Reoperation war der Patient 68 Jahre alt, die Lindenhof-Prothese links gerade 20 Jahre in situ. 18 Jahre lang war der Patient völlig beschwerdefrei und übte seinen Beruf als Winzer aus. Während der ganzen Zeit hat der Patient keine Kontrollen durchführen lassen. In den letzten beiden Jahren waren zunehmend belastungsabhängige Schmerzen im linken Hüftgelenk aufgetreten. Die Röntgenaufnahme vor der Reoperation (Abb. 1) zeigte eine Wanderung der Pfanne nach kranial und vor allem zentral, Trochanter major und Trochanter minor waren durch eine große Osteolyse um den zementierten Schaft fast völlig resorbiert. Bei der Operation entleerte sich massiv schwarzer trüber Erguß, das Gewebe der

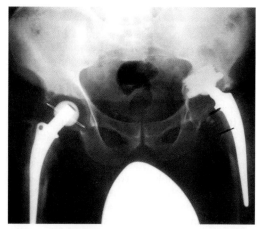

Abb. 1 Röntgenaufnahme Beckenübersicht 20 Jahre nach Lindenhofendoprothese links. Hochgradige Pfannenwanderung, proximales Drittel des zementierten Schaftes infolge Osteolyse freistehend.

Neokapselinnenhaut war schwarz, die Osteolysehöhle mit schwarzem nekrotische Detritus gefüllt. Nach Entfernung der im Becken verklemmten Keramikpfanne fand sich schwarzes Granulationsgewebe auch hinter dem Pfannenboden. Kopf (26 mm) und Pfannenloch zeigten massiven Abriebsubstanzverlust (< 3 mm, Abb. 2a), der kraniale Rand des Pfannenlochs zusätzlich, daß hier größere Keramikanteile abgeplatzt waren. Der in die Gelenkhöhle ragende Hals und die Halsauflage des CoCrMo-Guß-Schaftes waren vor allem im Schulterbereich grob zerkratzt, die ursprünglich kantigen Ränder der Halsauflage gerundet und poliert (Abb. 2b). Der Zementköcher des nicht gelockerten Schaftes war auch im Osteolysebereich noch intakt. Die histologische Untersuchung des aus allen Arealen entnommenen Granulationsgewebes zeigte überall die typischen Keramik-Kristalleinlagerungen mit Korngrößen $< = 5\,\mu$, die in Makrophagennestern, ganz vereinzelt als größere Splitter mit Fremdkörperriesenzellen assoziiert,

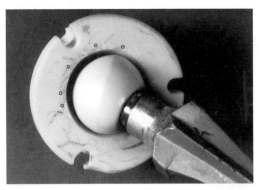 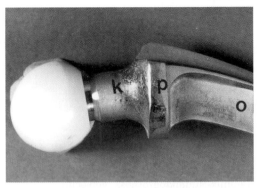

Abb. 2a Nahaufnahme des Explantates 20 Jahre post impl. Erhebl. Verschleiß von Keramikkopf und Keramikpfanne; Kreise markieren zusätzliche Abplatzdefekte am Verschleißrand der Pfanne.

Abb. 2b Nahaufnahme der Kopf-Hals-Region des CoCrMo-Guß-Schaftes. K = flächenhafte grob sichtbare Kratzdefekte an der Prothesenschulter; p = Polierabtrag des ursprünglich scharfkantigen proximalen Kragenrandes; 0 = unversehrte ursprüngliche Legierungsoberfläche.

die im Bindegewebe eingelagert waren. Meist jedoch fanden sich Mischgranulome, die Keramik- und hochfeinen Metallabrieb gemeinsam enthielten, dann auch mit stärkerer Rundzellreaktion. Diese Mischgranulome waren vor allem oberflächlich, d.h. gelenk- bzw. implantatnah konzentriert, während die reinen Keramikabriebnester bevorzugt in tieferen Gewebsschichten zu beobachten waren. Dies legt nahe, daß die Mischgranulome rezenteren Datums sind und den zeitlichen Ablauf des Verschleißprozesses widerspiegeln. Offenbar war das Gelenk über viele Jahre relativ stabil gewesen bis die Pfannenmigration einerseits und Abrieb andererseits zur Gelenkinkongruenz führten, so daß der gefürchtete Dreikörperabrieb den Verschleißprozeß exponentiell wachsen ließ. Die dann in größerer Menge im Gelenkraum anfallenden Keramikpartikel haben den nicht vom Zement geschützten in die Gelenkhöhle ragenden Teil des Metallschaftes zerkratzt und poliert mit nachfolgender massiver Metallose und den die Osteolyse fördernden Mischgranulomen. Der Vorgang ähnelt dem Läppen von Metallteilen mit Korundpulver in der Technik freilich in unserem Falle mit katastrophalen Folgen. Zementbestandteile haben wir histologisch nicht gefunden, so daß diese als Ursache ausscheiden.

Wie sollen wir uns also verhalten, wenn Keramik/Keramik-Prothesen im Patienten Probleme bereiten. Um diese rechtzeitig zu erkennen, müssen die Patienten regelmäßig klinisch und röntgenologisch vor allem langfristig kontrolliert werden. Am Besten geschieht dies durch die operierende Klinik, da niedergelassene Fachkollegen oder Röntgenologen mit der besonderen Problematik in der Regel nicht so vertraut sind. Stellungsänderungen der Pfanne und Osteolysen müssen frühzeitig erkannt und mit der Möglichkeit der beschriebenen besonderen Verschleiß-Situation in Verbindung gebracht werden. In kürzeren Kontrollabständen läßt sich dann die Dynamik des Geschehens beurteilen und die Reoperation zügig planen. Bei Bruch von Keramikkomponenten sollte so schnell wie möglich reoperiert werden. Da die komplette Entfernung des vorhandenen Keramikabriebs bei der Reoperation im Einzelfall nicht sicher möglich sein wird, können nur wiederum Keramik/Keramik-Gleitpartner eingesetzt werden, da alle anderen zur Verfügung stehenden Materialien in Verbindung mit Keramik-Partikeln im Gelenkspalt zu schnellem katastrophalem Verschleiß führen können (siehe hierzu auch 3). Wie die beschriebenen histologischen Untersuchungen zeigen, findet sich der Keramikabrieb an allen Grenzflächen der ersten Prothese, so daß im Zweifelsfalle alle auch festsitzende Komponenten gewechselt werden sollten, um das Implantatbett möglichst gründlich zu säubern. Besonders problematisch und diskussionswürdig ist weiterhin die Frage nach der Verankerung der neuen Prothese – zementiert oder zementfrei? Schmalzried et. al. (4) haben mit dem Konzept des „effective joint space" eindrücklich darstellen können, daß zementfrei verankerte Prothesen nie komplett und schlüssig einwachsen, so daß entlang der Verankerung im Knochen immer mikroskopische Spalten bleiben, die das Einwandern von Abriebpartikeln erlauben (siehe hierzu auch 2). Bei Reoperationen ist ein exakter Formschluß ohnehin meist nicht möglich, so daß vorbestehende Spalten zum Einwandern von verbliebenen Keramikabriebteilchen geradezu einladen. In Einzelfällen muß erneut mit Läppeffekten und Metallose gerechnet werden. Eine Zementierung der neuen Komponenten reduziert zwar die Problematik des sog. Effective joint space, wird jedoch aus anderen Gründen von der Mehrzahl der Operateure abgelehnt werden. Man wird wohl in Kenntnis der Gesamtproblematik von Fall zu Fall entscheiden müssen, welche Lösung die sicherste ist. Auch muß die künftige Erfahrung zu diesen Fragen zeigen, ob die diskutierten Problemkreise klinisch tatsächlich so relevant sind. Es wäre deshalb sinnvoll, Wechseloperationen mit Keramik/Keramikkomponenten zentral zu erfassen, um möglichst schnell an mehr Informationen zu kommen, die die Beantwortung der aufgeworfenen Fragen fördern.

Literaturhinweise

1. Griss, P., Hartz, U., Willert, H.-G. (1985): Analyse der periprothetischen Gewebereaktion bei 26 reoperierten Hüftendoprothesen der Al_2O_3-Keramik-Gleitpaarung. Z. Orthop. 668–669.
2. Griss, P., Fuchs, G. A., Franke, P. (1994): Die aggressive zystische Granulomatose des Femurschaftes – Polyaethylen – Krankheit als limitierender Faktor der Haltbarkeit zementfreier Hüftendoprothesenschäfte? Osteologie 3, 22–32.
3. Kempf, J., Semlitsch, M. (1990): Massive wear of a steel ball head by ceramic fragments in the polyethylene acetabular cup after revision of a total hip prosthesis with fractured ceramic ball. Arch. Orthop. Trauma Surg. 109, 284–287.
4. Schmalzried, T.P., Jasty, M., Harris, W.H.(1992): Periprosthetic bone loss in total hip arthroplasty – polyaethylene wear debris and the concept of effective joint space. J. Bone Jt. Surg. 74A, 849–863.

2.5 Revisionsstrategie bei der Verwendung von Keramikköpfen

M. Fröhling, L. Zichner, R. Koch

Nach wie vor stellt die Gleitpaarung Keramikkopf/ Polyethylenpfanne den Standard der modernen Hüftendoprothetik dar. Der Keramikkopf ist dabei über den sogenannten „Eurokonus", einen 10%-Konus, üblicherweise in der Dimensionierung 12/14, mit dem Hüftendoprothesenschaft verbunden. Die gleiche Metall-Keramik-Konusverbindung kommt im Rahmen der wachsenden Anzahl von Keramik-Keramik-Gleitpaarungen zur Anwendung.

Aufgrund einer rasch steigenden Anzahl von Wechseloperationen wegen aseptischer Hüftendoprothesenlockerung muß eine große Anzahl von Keramikköpfen auf dem verbleibenden Hüftendoprothesenschaft ausgetauscht werden, wenn dieser noch fest ist und deshalb nicht gewechselt wird. Es stellt sich dabei die Frage, ob der Keramikkopf gegen einen weiteren Keramikkopf oder aber gegen einen Metallkopf gewechselt werden sollte.

Die Hersteller beantworten diese Frage mit einem klaren nein, da Labormessungen ergeben haben, daß die Bruchfestigkeit eines auf denselben Konus gewechselten Keramikkopfes um 30% reduziert ist.

Für diesen Standpunkt sprechen auch die belastungsbedingten morphologischen Veränderungen des Metallkonus, der, um sich der viel härteren Keramik im Sinne einer dauerhaft festen Verbindung anpassen zu können, über eine feine Ril-

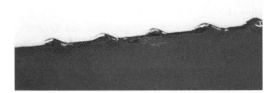

Abb. 2 Mikroskopisches Bild der deformierten Rillenstruktur eines „Eurokonus" nach Belastung durch das Körpergewicht.

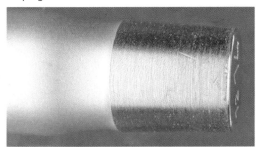

Abb. 3

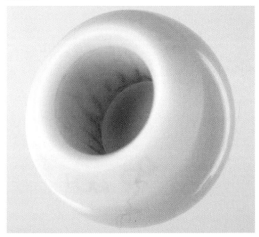

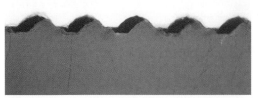

Abb. 1 Mikroskopisches Bild der intakten Rillenstruktur eines „Eurokonus".

Abb. 3 und 4 Kraftübertragungszone von Kopf und Schaftkonus nach Belastung.

lenstruktur verfügt (Abb. 1). Wird diese Rillenstruktur belastet, verformt sie sich im Sinne einer Anpassung an die härtere Keramik (Abb. 2). Dadurch wird die kraftübertragende Fläche in Richtung Konusbasis vergrößert (Abb. 3 und 4).

Dabei wird das Ziel verfolgt, den Keramikkopf zunächst in seinem Zentrum und nicht in der Konuseingangsebene zu belasten, in der er bezüglich einer möglichen Sprengwirkung besonders vulnerabel ist. Erreicht wird dieser regelhaft ablaufende Vorgang durch einen, verglichen mit dem Konuswinkel des Schaftes, einen bis wenige Winkelminuten größeren Konuswinkel des Kopfkonus. Einen Hauptgrund für diese Vorgehensweise stellen produktionstechnisch nicht zu vermeidende Fertigungstoleranzen dar, die theoretisch zu einer bevorzugten Belastung der Konuseingangsebene führen könnten.

Ist nun eine Konusverbindung belastet worden und hat dadurch eine Deformation der Rillenstruktur erfahren, so ist dieser Anpassungsprozeß nicht oder zumindest nicht mehr im gleichen Maße möglich. Theoretisch kann dies zu einer stärkeren Belastung in der Konuseingangsebene des Keramikkopfes führen. Praktisch führt es im Laborbelastungsversuch zu der o.g. reduzierten Bruchfestigkeit des Keramikkopfes.

Die beschriebene reduzierte Bruchfestigkeit, die Herstellerempfehlungen sowie nicht zuletzt haftungsrechtliche Überlegungen begründen die Kopfwechselstrategie der Orthopädischen Universitätsklinik Frankfurt. Dabei sind folgende unterschiedliche Ausgangssituationen zu unterscheiden:

1. Wechsel des Keramikkopfes während der Primäroperation zur Veränderung der Beinlänge oder des lateralen Offsets, ohne daß der Kopf durch das Körpergewicht belastet wurde: In dieser Situation ist ein Wechsel Keramik/Keramik möglich, da eine Deformation der Rillenstruktur des Schaftkonus nicht stattgefunden hat. Voraussetzung dabei ist, daß sich der Primärkopf nicht auf dem Schaftkonus verkeilt hat und sich leicht entfernen läßt.
2. Wird der Keramikkopf im Rahmen einer Revisionoperation, d. h. nach Belastung durch das Körpergewicht, gewechselt, so ist aufgrund der abgelaufenen Deformation der Rillenstruktur des Schaftkonus der Wechsel auf einen Metallkopf erforderlich.
3. Ist anläßlich einer Wechseloperation der Kopf gelockert, so liegt eine, in der Regel auch makroskopisch sichtbare, schwerwiegende Defor-

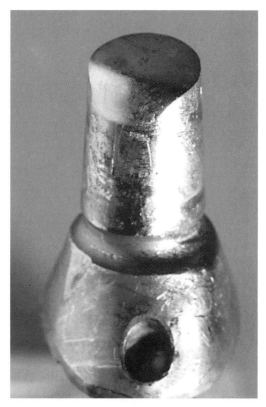

Abb. 5 Abradierter Schaftkonus nach Keramikkopffraktur und Kopfwechsel ohne Schaftwechsel.

mation des Schaftkonus vor, die neben dem Kopf- auch einen Schaftwechsel erfordert.
4. Bei frakturiertem Keramikkopf ist ebenfalls der Schaftkonus genau auf Beschädigungen zu untersuchen und aufgrund schwerwiegender Beschädigungen in der Regel zu wechseln (Abb. 5). Insbesondere muß jedoch das Polyethyleninlay der Pfanne gewechselt werden, da sich Splitter des frakturierten Keramikkopfes in das Polyethylen der Pfanne imprimieren und den neuen Kopf abradieren (Abb. 6 und 7), was im Falle eines Metallkopfes zu einer ausgeprägten Metallose führt.

Da sich die Keramiksplitter eines frakturierten Kopfes auch in den periartikulären Weichteilen befinden und aus diesen nicht zuverlässig entfernt werden können, ist zu diskutieren, ob in diesem Fall unter Inkaufnahme der reduzierten Bruchfestigkeit auf einen Keramikkopf gewechselt werden sollte.

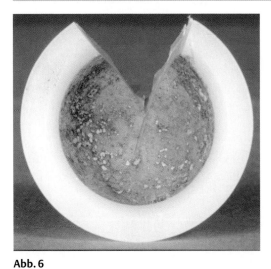 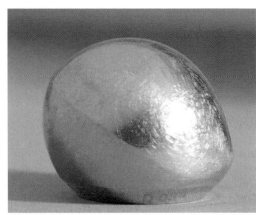

Abb. 6   **Abb. 7**

Abb. 6 und 7 Kopfabrasion durch in die Polyethylenpfanne imprimierte Keramiksplitter nach Keramikkopffraktur und Wechsel auf einen Metallkopf ohne gleichzeitigen Inlaywechsel.

2.6 Revision Strategy for Ceramic Implant Failures

L. Sedel

Revision of a total hip made totally or partially of alumina ceramics is not very different from regular hip revision. However there are some special features that must be known by the orthopaedic surgeon who will perform the revision. It is these specific problems or issues that we would like to address here.

As alumina on alumina provides few debris, reasons for revisions are rather different than those for regular material.

Reasons are usually not related to osteolysis or poor bone support but to either material fracture, mechanical aseptic loosening of acetabular component with good bone support, recurrent dislocation, some impingement problems that could resume in metallic debris, and also some unexplained pain, as regular total hip. Lack of osteolysis permitted usually to perform a limited revision, leaving the femoral component in place. The limited wear of ceramics component allotted sometimes revision that retain even the ceramic head and sometimes in our experience that will only resume in cementing a cementless alumina ceramics component.

Lets look at these different situations.

Fracture

We have to separate acute fracture or fracture that did evolve slowly with a initial crack that will progress; some histories we have recorded to fall in this category; For example in our series, the only fracture of an alumina linner occured in a 59 years old woman who was operated in 1992. Results was excellent; In 1994 she sustained a car accident and was again operated in our department for a patella fracture on the side of the total hip. At this time, clinical and radiological evaluation of the hip were considered as perfect. During the year 1997 she was revised on the same hip for groin pain, images of osteolysis on the X rays; The surgeon documented the revision, the liner was fractured and displaced leaving some ceramic on metal friction to occur; this explains the osteolysis and the pain; Then we can suspect the fracture of the patella to be concomitant with a ceramic liner crack initiation that slowly did evolve to a complete fracture.

When a fracture of ceramics occurred we can suspect many debris of different size to be generated in the articulation; Then when we have to revise, the surgeon must be aware of taking out all the debris but also to take into consideration that as it is never possible to clear totally the operating field, he will have to use special material to replace the hip .Metallic head must be avoided because the remaining ceramic debris could be trapped into the polyethylene of the socket and give rise to very severe damaged of the metallic head as reported by Kempf and others ( ). Then it is absolutely necessary to use another ceramic head either in a ceramic on ceramic couple either in a ceramic on polyethylene.

If the Morse taper has been damaged because of the long term fracture, it has to be replaced. If it is a case of acute fracture quickly revised, the cone is usually not damaged and another ceramic head could be fixed on the old taper; This will avoid femoral stem revision which is by far a difficult procedure.

Mechanical loosening

In this circumstances there can be many different situation:

The first one is when the mechanical loosening occurred acutely or even slowly. In the first condition, there are very few debris; many papers demonstrated that wear in regular situation is very low, then we can expect very few debris, and also very limited wear of the component's surface; then it can be possible to retain the same head and even the same socket; for example in some of bulky alumina loosening, we retained the same socket that was cemented. If the socket has been loosed for a long time and had tilted, we have to replace the acetabular sliding surface; If the head has not been damaged, we can retain the same head, and replace the acetabular by another ceramic material with a metal backed or if the patient is older than 65 or 70 by a plain polyethylene socket cemented.

If the cone had been badly damaged, or if, due to impingement, the femoral stem presents some rubbing marks, it is better to exchange the stem for another one. And then still use at least one sliding component (the head) made of alumina ceramics.

How to deal with a cone that had already received a ceramic head.

Due to cone technology, the cone is theoretically damaged and the engineers will advise to replace the cone as well if a new ceramic head has to be implanted; The other solution could be to use a metallic head. But, as we know from different report, the risk of putting a metallic head after retrieval of ceramic component is very high of getting a severe metallic wear with massive abrasion and need to revision in short term period.

Practically there are three situations:
- there is a mechanical loosening of the socket, which did not tilt, we exchange the socket sometimes without exchanging the head or sometimes, for technical reasons, we take out the head during the revision and put it back at the end. We check that the fixation is secure.
- there is a mechanical loosening of the socket with some impingement or tilting of the socket; Usually the head in this situation could have been worn out; Then it is better to exchange the socket and the head; If the cone looks good, we check the fixation of the new head on the cone; If this seems secure, we retain this solution; If not, we exchange the stem as well, putting another ceramic head on the taper.
- there is a mechanical loosening of both components, reconstruction is conducted in a regular way, but always a ceramic head has to be utilized sliding either on a ceramic acetabulum if the patient is young or very active, or a polyethylene socket if not.

In case we put another ceramic head on the same Morse taper, we have to explain to the patient that there is an increased risk of alumina ceramic fracture. We did that in 29 cases over 61 revisions performed in a series of 401 hips. These patients were followed very accurately and none of them sustained a ceramic head fracture in the following period up to 15 years.

Conclusion

Revision strategy when we have to retrieve alumina ceramics material must be precise. Surgeon must be aware of the specificity of this material: very limited wear and no osteolysis in regular situation which allow sometimes to implant the same components, risk of ceramics debris in the surrounding tissues that could eventually badly damage a metallic head if implanted instead of the ceramic one, risk of fracture of the ceramic head if implanted on a Morse taper that already had a ceramic head.

We tried in this short paper to explain the way to overcome these situations and how we can deal with. Surgeons and engineers could have some different strategies, the answer are always, as in every surgery, in the calculated risk of each situation.

References

1. Kempf I, Semlith M. Massive wear of a steel ball head by ceramic fragments in the polyethylene acetabular cup after revision of a total hip prosthesis with fractured ceramic ball. Arch Orthop Trauma Surg 1990, 109(5): 284–287.
2. Sedel L., Bizot P., Nizard R., Meunier A. Perspective on a 25 years experience with ceramic on ceramic articulation in total hip replacement. Seminars in arthroplasty vol 9, N°2, 1998, 123–134
3. Hip Surgery materials and development. Laurent Sedel et Miguel Cabanela. Ed. Martin Dunitz London. 1998.

3 Reliability – Technical Aspects

3.1 Wear and Debris Generation in Artificial Hip Joints

J. Fisher, E. Ingham, M.H. Stone, B.M. Wroblewski, P.S.M. Barbour, A.A. Besong, J.L. Tipper, J.B. Matthews, P.J. Firkins, A.B. Nevelos, J.E. Nevelos

Introduction

Over the last thirty years the majority of artificial hip joints used clinically have utilised ultra high molecular weight polyethylene UHMWPE as the bearing surface of the acetabular cup. Although these bearing surfaces rarely wear out and indeed provide a very effective solution for the elderly patient, it is now recognised that in the longer term, micron and submicron UHMWPE wear particles generated at the articulating surfaces, lead to chronic inflammatory tissue reactions, osteolysis and loosening of the prostheses. This has led to renewed interest in metal on metal and ceramic on ceramic bearing couples. There is now a real need to focus attention, not just on the wear volume generated, but also the actual wear particles produced and their osteolytic potential. In this paper, research studies from our laboratory are reviewed which quantify the wear and wear debris generated in hip joint simulators and are compared to data from retrieved prostheses, for metal and ceramic on UHMWPE, metal on metal and ceramic on ceramic bearing couples.

Methods

The Leeds physiological hip joint simulators have six degrees of freedom and test the prostheses in the anatomical position. The Mark 1 simulator has independently controlled forces, applied to three axes and three independently controlled motions (4). The force and motion wave forms are applied as defined in the Paul walking cycle. It has been shown that for UHMWPE acetabular cups simplification of the loading cycle to a single axis of loading does not substantially alter the wear rate (3). The Mark 2 simulator has one axis of loading and two independently controlled motions (2). This has been shown to produce volumetric wear rates for UHMWPE acetabular cups equivalent to the Mark 1 simulator.

The results of tests carried out on size 28 mm metal and ceramic heads on UHMWPE cups, size 28 mm, metal on metal, and size 28 mm Ceramtec Biolox Forte ceramic on ceramic hips are reviewed. The analysis of debris is presented from metal and ceramic on UHMWPE and from metal on metal hip prostheses and a comparison is made with clinical retrievals.

Results

Metal and Ceramic Heads on UHMWPE Acetabular Cups

Ultrahigh molecular weight polyethylene UHMWPE acetabular cups that were gamma irradiated in the presence of air and tested within three years of sterilisation were studied. Stainless steel, cobalt chrome and zirconia femoral heads were tested in the Mark 1 and Mark 2 simulators for 5 million cycles. The volumetric wear rates are presented in Table (1). There was a statistically significant difference in the wear rates with the different heads.

These volumetric wear rates were compared with a clinical series of retrieved Charnley hip prostheses that had failed by aseptic loosening.

Table 1 Volumetric wear rates for UHMWPE acetabular cups

Material			Volumetric Wear
Head	Cup	Simulator	mm³ per million cycles ± 95% CL
Stainless Steel	UHMWPE	Mark 2	41 ± 4
Cobalt Chrome	UHMWPE	Mark 2	35 ± 10
Zirconia	UHMWPE	Mark 2	31 ± 4
Zirconia	UHMWPE	Mark 1	32 ± 3.4

The mean age of these prostheses was 13 years range (10 to 19) and the prostheses had 22 mm stainless steel femoral heads with UHMWPE cups that had been γ irradiated in air (10). The mean volumetric wear rate (± 95% CL) was 59.6 ± 17.9 mm³/year. There was substantial variation in the wear rates. The group was further analysed by dividing into two groups of explants, one with low damage to the femoral head and one with high damage to the femoral head. The low damage group had a significantly lower wear rate, which was comparable to the wear caused by the undamaged heads in the simulator (Table 2).

Table 2 Volumetric wear rates for explanted Charnley prostheses (10)

Material	Volumetric Wear Rate	
	mm³/year	± 95% CL
Low damaged heads	39.5	± 22.6
High damaged heads	79.6	± 21.2

Difference significant at the 93% level

The polyethylene wear debris was isolated and characterised from the Mark 1 simulator test. The particles were primarily micron or submicron in size. The quantitative analysis of the particles is summarised in Table (3).

Table 3 Quantification of wear debris from hip simulator (mean ± 95% CL)

Mode of the particle size distribution	0.1 to 0.5 μm
% Mass of particles < 10 μm	73 ± 6
Number of particles per mm³ x 10⁹	35 ± 25
Volumetric wear rate per million cycles mm³	32 ± 3.4
Number of particles per million cycles x 10⁹	1100

The UHMWPE debris from the retrieved tissues showed considerable similarity to the debris from the simulator, although there was greater variation and some important differences. The mode of the particle size distribution and the percentage mass of the debris which was less than 10 μm, were similar. However, there were less particles in the very small size range in the retrieved tissues compared to the simulator debris, possibly due to them being transported away *in vivo* and lost from the analysis. This resulted in a calculation of less particles per mm³ of debris resulting in less particles per year. The explant debris data are summarised in Table 4.

Table 4 Wear debris analysis for explanted tissue mean ± 95% CL (10)

Mode of the particle size distribution	0.1 to 0.5 μm
% Mass of particles < 10 ± μm in size	68 ± 15
Number of particles per mm³ x 10⁹	13.2 ± 9.6
Mean volumetric wear rate mm³/year	59.6 ± 17.8
Number of particles generated per year x 10⁹	496

In addition to an increase in the volumetric wear, damage to the femoral head of the explanted prostheses also significantly increased the number of UHMWPE wear particles generated.

Metal on Metal Hip Prostheses

Six metal on metal hip prostheses were tested in the Leeds Mark 1 physiological simulator for up to 5 million cycles. The cobalt chrome alloys consisted of two pairs of low carbon content alloys, two pairs of high carbon content alloys and two pairs of mixed alloys (low carbon head and high carbon cup).

The volumetric wear rates are shown in Table (5). They were all much lower than found with UHMWPE. All the prostheses showed a higher initial bedding in wear followed by a lower steady state wear. The mixed and high carbon pairings showed lower wear than in the low carbon pairing (5). Clinical studies have reported higher volumetric wear rates with first generation McKee Farrar Prostheses (1).

Table 5 Volumetric wear rates for metal on metal hip prostheses (5)

Material	Volumetric wear mm³/year per million cycles		
	Average	Initial	Steady State
High Carbon Alloy	0.09	0.32	0.03
Mixed Carbon Alloy	0.09	0.31	0.03
Low Carbon Alloy	0.51	1.36	0.33

The metal debris was isolated from the serum and quantified using SEM. The resolution of the measurement system was 10 nm. The metal debris was much smaller than the polyethylene debris and more uniform in size and shape (see Table 6).

Table 6 Particle sizes of metal on metal debris (5)

Material	Particle Size nm	
	Mean	±95% CL
High Carbon Alloy	36	±2
Mixed Carbon Alloy	25	±1
Low Carbon Alloy	25	±1

For the high carbon content alloy, taking a mean size of 36 nm and a spherical geometry the mean size of a particle was estimated as $0.24 \, 10^5$ (nm)^3. The estimate of the number of particles generated is presented in Table (7).

Table 7 Estimated number of particles per year for metal-on-metal prostheses

Number of particles per mm^3	$4.2 \, 10^{13}$
Volumetric wear rate mm^3/million cycles	0.09
Number of particles per million cycles	$4 \, 10^{12}$

Although the volumetric wear rate was 100 times less than UHMWPE, the number of particles generated per million cycles was greater due to the particles being much smaller in size. It should be noted however that the detection level for metal particles was lower than for UHMWPE.

Ceramic on Ceramic Hip Prostheses

Six Biolox Forte alumina alumina hip prostheses were tested in the Mark 2 Leeds Physiological simulator. After two million cycles, the angle of inclination of four of the cups was increased from 45° to 60°. This did not, however, alter the wear rate. The cups showed a higher initial bedding-in wear rate then a lower steady state wear rate (9). The volumetric wear rate is shown in Table (8).

The steady state wear rate was similar to that achieved with metal on metal prostheses and three orders of magnitude lower than achieved with UHMWPE.

Table 8 Volumetric wear rates for Biolox Forte Hips (9)

Material Biolox Forte	Volumetric Wear Rate mm^3/million cycles	±95% CL
Initial Wear	0.12	±0.6
Steady State Wear Rate	0.05	±0.02

Clinical wear rates with Mittelmeier Biolox prostheses have been reported as greater in certain cases of stripe and severe wear (8). Debris has not been characterised from the simulator tests. However, there was very little surface disruption indicating very fine debris, perhaps in the order of 10 nm with this very low wear. In the more severe wear cases found clinically with Biolox ceramic, the wear surfaces were rougher with fragments of grains removed and evidence of larger debris in the size range 0.1 to 5 µm (8).

Discussion

The volumetric wear rates in the simulators showed a clear ranking with UHMWPE being greater than metal on metal or Biolox Forte alumina ceramic. There was good agreement between the simulation volumetric wear rates and clinical retrievals for UHMWPE, but for metal on metal and ceramic on ceramic, the simulators produced lower wear rates than found *in vivo*. This may be due to the clinical retrievals being different older types or inferior materials, or possibly due to the more adverse conditions that can occur *in vivo*.

The UHMWPE debris produced was predominantly in the 0.1 to 10 µm size range. This size range has been shown to be highly biologically reactive in activating macrophages and causing bone resorption (6, 7). There is evidence that very small UHMWPE particles (<0.5 µm) are transported away form the prosthesis and surrounding tissues. The metal particles were much smaller than the UHMWPE particles. Although there were a greater number of the smaller metal particles generated, compared to UHMWPE, the total number of metal particles produced in the size range that caused high levels of biological reactivity for UHMWPE (0.1 to 10 µm) was much lower than for UHMWPE. As a result of the different sizes, chemical activity and ion release, the metal particles are likely to be distributed more widely around the body and cause different biological reactions. These biological reactions to small metal particles are currently being studied.

There is limited understanding of the types of ceramic debris produced. The evidence presented so far indicates that for very low wear conditions, very small particles may be produced but with more severe wear as found with older Biolox ceramic larger particles in the size range 0.1 to 10 µm, a similar size to that of UHMWPE, can be found. The biological reactions and distribution *in vivo* will be dependent on size, and this needs to be studied further. The clinical evidence with the Biolox ceramic Mittlemeir prosthesis indicates that as the volume of wear was much smaller than with UHMWPE, the resulting number of particles in the biologically active size range (0.1 to 10 μm) was much less and the occurrence of osteolysis was reduced considerably (8).

Conclusions

The reduction in wear volumes with alternate bearing surfaces to UHMWPE, provides considerable potential for extending the osteolysis free life of artificial hip joints beyond 20 years. However, the size of the wear particles varies considerably for the different materials. Future research will focus on the performance of new bearing designs under adverse conditions, on quantifying the size, number and the biological activity of the different wear particles.

Acknowledgement

This work was supported in part by The Arthritis Research Campaign, The John Charnley Trust, Department of Trade and Industry, Engineering Physical Science Research Council, Johnson & Johnson DePuy and Howmedica International.

References

1. Amstutz HC, Grigoris P. Metal on metal bearings in hip arthroplasty. Clinical Orthopaedics and Related Research, 3295, 511–34, 1996.
2. Barbour PSM, Stone MH, Fisher J. A hip joint simulator study using simplified loading and motion cycles generating physiological wear particles and wear rates. J. Eng. in Med. (*in press*).
3. Besong AA, Bigsby RJA, Barbour PSM, Fisher J. Effect of head size and loading regime on UHMWPE cup wear. Proc. World Tribology Congress, 732, 1997.
4. Bigsby RJA, Hardaker CS, Fisher J. Wear of UHMWPE in a physiological hip joint simulator in the anatomical position. J. Eng. in Med. 211, 265–269, 1997.
5. Firkins PJ, Tipper JL, Farrar R, Stone MH, Ingham E, Fisher J. Quantitative analysis of wear debris from metal on metal hip prostheses tested in a physiological simulator. Trans 45th ORS, 24, 1999.
6. Green TR, Fisher J, Stone MH, Wroblewski BM, Ingham E. Polyethylene particles of a critical size are necessary for induction of cytokines by macrophages. Biomaterials 19, 2297–2302, (1998).
7. Green TR, Matthews JB, Fisher J, Ingham E. Polyethylene particles of a critical size are necessary for the induction of TNF_α by macrophages *in vitro*. Trans. 44th ORS, 23, 1998.
8. Nevelos JN, Ingham E, Doyle C, Nevelos AB, Fisher J. Examination of alumina ceramic components from Mittlemeier total hip arthroplasties. Trans. 44th ORS, 23, 219, 1998.
9. Nevelos JN, Ingham E, Doyle C, Fisher J. Influence of acetabular cup angle on the wear of Biolox Forte alumina/alumina hip joints in a physiological simulator. Trans. 45th ORS, 24, 1999.
10. Tipper JL, Ingham E, Besong AA, Wroblewski BM, Stone MH, Fisher J. Quantitative comparison of polyethylene wear debris, wear rate and head damage in retrieved Charnley hip prostheses. J. Mat. Sci. Materials in Medicine (*in press*).

3.2 New Wear Couples for THR – Simulator Testing

A. Toni, S. Affatato

Abstract

Wear of hip implants is a significant clinical problem. In prosthetic hip surgery polyethylene wear is indicated as a factor that limits the duration of the implant; the limitation of wear is of fundamental to the optimisation of THR longevity.

Two types of mixed oxides ceramic femoral heads and acetabular cups containing different ratios of alumina and zirconia were compared with pure commercial alumina in terms of wear behaviour in a hip joint simulator.

Mixed oxides ceramics have been indicated in literature as a promising compromise between strength and wear but no reports are available on the influence of a percentage of zirconia in a ceramic femoral head when sliding against itself. Mixed oxides ceramic acetabular cups and femoral heads were tested on a simulator apparatus with a sinusoidal load in presence of bovine calf serum. The experimental results have shown no significant difference between the experimental and commercial ceramic material couplings.

Introduction

Ceramic is a class of new engineering materials for wear resistant applications under severe environments. Ceramics materials for total hip replacement (THR) were introduced more than 20 years ago (1).

In recent years ceramic materials have been recognized as being increasing by important for their chemical and physical characteristics, and have progressively attracted interest in the field of biomedicine (2,3). The ceramic materials most frequently used as constituents of prosthetic components are alumina and zirconia (4). Alumina ceramics have been widely used for their thermomechanical, and tribologic properties (5). Zirconia ceramics have been introduced as an alternative to alumina, being used as the material of the modular femoral head in total hip replacement joint (6).

It is widely accepted that for any biomedical device it is generally difficult to combine in one material all the properties required for excellence in functionality, tribological behaviour and biocompatibility. As a result, compromise may have to be made or combinations of two or more materials used to develop the best overall properties. A good solution to this dilemma was achieved adding two different fractions of zirconia to alumina to obtain a new class of materials.

Therefore, alumina and a variable fraction of zirconia, were tested and compared with pure commercial alumina. This paper describes the tribological behaviour of these ceramic materials using a hip joint simulator.

Tests were carried out up to 10 million cycles since it is essential to validate, for long periods, materials used in prosthetic hip implants, in order to acquire further knowledge about their tribological behaviour and reduce the risk of clinical implant failure *in vivo*.

Materials and Methods

The materials used in the present study consisted of 32 mm diameter as follows:
- four 100% commercially available alumina ball heads and acetabular cups (ref. **0Zr**);
- four experimental 40% alumina-60% zirconia ball heads and acetabular cups (ref. **60Zr**);
- four experimental 20% alumina-80% zirconia ball heads and acetabular cups (ref. **80Zr**).

The pure alumina ball heads and acetabular cups (ref. **0Zr**) used in the present study were supplied by Officine Ortopediche Rizzoli (Bologna-Italy) and are commercial products available on the market as Biolox Forte (CeramTec, Germany). The eight mixed-oxides ball heads and acetabular cups, were manufactured in-house. The manufacturing process was developed by Centro Ceramico

(Bologna – Italy) and by FN S.p.A. (Bosco Marengo – Italy).

The wear test was conducted using a twelve stations hip joint wear simulator (Shore Western, U.S.A.). In the hip joint simulator the heads were mounted using self-aligning connection components while the cups were fixed to a titanium holder and mounted on a bearing block to represent the natural flexion angle between cup and hip joint load axis. The load profile was sinusoidal with peak magnitude of 2030 N and a frequency of 1 Hz. The rotation test frequency was about 70 cycles per minute with inversion between clockwise and counter clockwise rotation every 5 hours.

The stations were filled with lubricant in order to wet completely the specimeńs contact surfaces. The lubricant used was 30% sterile bovine calf serum (SIGMA, St. Louis, USA) and 70% deionised water plus 0.2% sodium azide (E. Merck, Darmstadt, Germany) to retard bacterial degradation during the wear test.

In the present work the wear was calculated by the weight loss method using a microbalance (SARTORIUS AG, Germany) with a sensitivity of 0.01 mg and an uncertainty of ± 0.10 mg.

The volumetric wear trend was evaluated in terms of weight loss *vs* number of load cycles taking into account of the polyethylene density and of wear rate *vs* number of load cycles. The wear rate was calculated at fixed intervals (every 500,000 cycles) as the weight loss since the previous interval over the number of cycles in the interval concerned. In the conversion of the weight loss into the vomuletric wear it was assumed that:
- 1 million cycles in the simulator represent a 1 year average *in vivo* activity (7);
- the density is 3.97, 5.02, and 5.49 mg/mm^3 for the **0Zr**, **60Zr** and **80Zr** compositions, respectively.

Results

The specimens completed the planned ten million cycles.

No damage was observed on either the cups or on the heads after 10 million cycles.

The evolution of wear for all four types of ceramic heads is plotted in Figure 1.

At 10 million cycles pure alumina acetabular cups showed a mean wear rate of $1.8 \cdot 10^{-5}$ mm * year^{-1}. The mixed-oxides acetabular cups showed a mean wear rate of $4.1 \cdot 10^{-5}$ mm · year^{-1} and $6.2 \cdot 10^{-5}$ mm · year^{-1} for the 80Zr and 60Zr composition respectively.

A non-parametric analysis (Kruskall-Wallis test) was performed to examine the statistical behaviour of the specimens. No significant differences were observed between all specimens tested in this study at a 95% level of confidence.

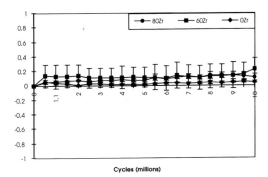

Fig. 1 Volumetric wear trend (mm^3)

Table 1 Characteristic of mixed oxides ceramic materials *vs* ISO-6474 and *vs* commercial alumina.

Characteristics		ISO 6474/94	80Zr	60Zr	0Zr (9)
Density	[g/cm^3]	≥ 3.94	5.49	5.02	3.97
Mean grain size	[mm]	≤ 4.5	Al$_2$O$_3$ = 0.38 ZrO$_2$ = 0.31	Al$_2$O$_3$ = 0.27 ZrO$_2$ = 0.50	< 2
Modulus of elasticity	[GPa]	–	259	285	380
Hardness	[GPa]	–	15.3 [HV$_{20}$]	15.1 [HV$_{20}$]	20 [HV$_{0.1}$]
Bending strength	[MPa]	–	1008	912	> 500
Fracture toughness	[MPa$\sqrt{m}$]	–	5.49	6.9	4

Discussions and Conclusions

Ceramic is a solid material with a crystalline structure containing no metallic element (8). This general definition includes many materials, only a few of which are used in the field of medicine for their chemical and physical properties. Two of the most frequently ceramics used in THR are alumina and zirconia. These materials present excellent biocompatibility (they are chemically stable being elements at the highest state of oxidation), and they have good properties of mechanical resistance and high wettability (3).

Mixtures of different percentages of alumina and zirconia were tried in order to obtain a ceramic material with the same tribological properties of alumina but with an improvement in mechanical properties. This potential new class of ceramics, partially stabilised zirconia, exhibit promising performances in relation to their toughness and extremely low surface roughness. The mechanical properties of the new class of ceramic materials are very attractive compared with the standard (Table 1).

Good *in vitro* wear results of ceramic on ceramic have been reported in this study. The results confirm that the tribological behaviour of experimental mixed oxides ceramic compares well with commercially pure alumina. The findings in this study permit us to conclude that experimental mixed oxides ceramic is a material of the future for hip implants. Being tribologically suitable for the femoral heads and acetabular cups of the total hip replacement joints, these new experimental mixed oxides ceramic materials could be an outstanding solution for orthopaedic applications.

References

1. Willmann G (1998) Ceramics for total hip replacement; what a surgeon should know. Orthopedics 21: 173–177
2. Cuckler JM, Bearcroft J, Asgian CM (1995) Femoral head technologies to reduce poliethylene wear in total hip arthroplasty. Clin Orthop 317: 57–63
3. Toni A, Terzi S, Sudanese A, Tabarroni M, Zappoli FA, Stea S, Giunti A (1995) The use of ceramic in prosthetic hip surgery. The state of the art. Chir. Organi Mov. LXXX: 13–25
4. Kumar P, Oka M, Ikeuchi K, Shimizu K, Yamamuro T, Okumura H, Koloura Y (1991) Low wear rates of UHMWPE against zirconia ceramic in comparison to alumina ceramic and SUS 316 alloy. J. Biomed. Mat. Res. 25: 813–828
5. McKellop H, Lu B (1992) Friction lubrication and wear of polyethylene metal and polyethylene ceramic hip prostheses in a joint simulator. Fourth World Biomaterials Congress, Berlin.
6. Esposito L, Tucci A (1997) Microstructural dependence of friction and wear behaviours in low purity alumina ceramics. Wear 205: 88–96
7. Saikko VO, Paavolainen PO, Slatis P (1993) Wear of the polyethylene acetabular cup: metallic and ceramic heads comparated in a hip simulator. Acta Orthop Scand 64: 391–402
8. Yammamuro T, Kotoua Y, Nakamura T, Kabutani Y, Kitsugi T (1989) Rationales for orthopaedic application of bioceramics. In: H. Oonishi, Aoki and K. Sawai (Eds), Bioceramics (Proceedings of 1st International Bioceramic Symposium), Kyto, Japan Vol. I: 19–24
9. Früh HJ, Willmann G (1998) Tribological investigations of the wear couple alumina-CFRP for total hip replacement. Biomaterials 19: 1145–1150

3.3 In-vitro Wear Performance of a Contemporary Alumina : Alumina Bearing Couple Under Anatomically-Relevant Hip Joint Simulation

S.K. Taylor

Purpose

The purpose of this study was to investigate the wear performance of a contemporary alumina:-alumina bearing couple versus CoCr:UHMWPE under hip joint simulation with an anatomically-relevant (i.e., superior cup) specimen orientation.

Test Articles

Alumina : Alumina

The alumina (Al_2O_3) components, shown in Figure 1, were produced by CeramTec (Plochingen Germany) and were certified as being produced from the Biolox® Forte alumina grade.

Femoral bearings were 28 mm in diameter with a +0 mm neck extension. Acetabular inserts were of the CeramTec XLW-18 design, with a nominal 39 mm outer diameter. Based on diameter and circularity tolerances specified in their respective drawings, the radial clearance between the alumina bearings and inserts ranged from 20–60 μm.

All ceramic test articles were exposed to 2.5–4.0 Mrad dosage gamma-irradiation sterilization prior to testing.

CoCr : UHMWPE

CoCr femoral bearings, 28 mm diameter, +0 mm neck extension, were obtained in their commercially-available condition.

UHMWPE acetabular inserts, 28 mm diameter with a 9.4 mm wall thickness, were machined from ram-extruded polyethylene (Poly Hi Solidur, Fort Wayne, IN, using Hoechst Celanese GUR 4150HP resin) consistent with ASTM F 648 (1), Type 2 requirements. Polyethylene inserts were also obtained in their as-commercially-available condition, which included nitrogen/vacuum packaging and gamma-irradiation sterilization. In order to reduce the effects of fluid absorption on wear measurements, polyethylene test articles were pre-soaked in room temperature distilled water for 30 days prior to testing.

All CoCr and UHMWPE test articles, included in Figure 1, were produced by Howmedica Osteonics (Allendale, N.J.)

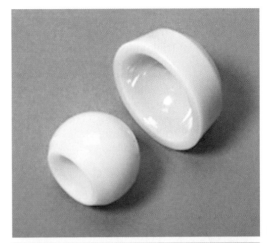
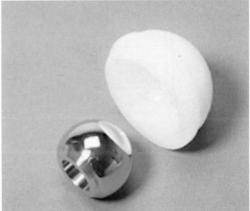

Fig. 1a,b a) Alumina : alumina test articles, b) CoCr : UHMWPE test articles.

Test Methods

Wear Exposure

Acetabular insert specimens were mounted in polyurethane molds housed in individual chambers, as shown in the test schematic in Figure 2. Four each of the alumina:alumina and CoCr: UHMWPE wear couples were subject to hip joint simulation under the following conditions:

Max. Load:	2500 N (562 lbs)
Waveform:	Paul (2) walking curve
Frequency:	1.0 Hz
Media:	Triple-filtered bovine calf serum with 0.1% sodium azide, 20 mM EDTA, 30% distilled water
Temperature:	Ambient (Note: Media temperature is typically 30–35°C due to system heating, but not controlled by design.)
Test Duration:	5×10^6 cycles

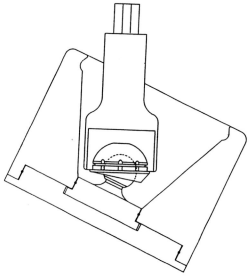

Fig. 2 Joint simulation test schematic on the MTS Multi-Station Hip Simulator.

The use of diluted serum has become increasingly accepted by the tribological community and dilution below 40% water content has been qualified for use in hip simulation (3).

Serum was continually replenished with distilled water to account for evaporation. Wear progressed 24 hrs/day for six days between weighings. The entire serum bath within each chamber was replaced every three days.

An MTS Multi-Station Hip Simulator (MTS Systems Corp., Eden Prairie, MN) was used to control load, waveform, and frequency.

Gravimetric Wear Measurement

Prior to wear exposure, the cup inserts were cleaned and weighed in triplicate, employing a Mettler Model AE 163 Dual Range Precision Balance (Mettler Instrument Corp., Hightstown, N.J.). UHMWPE inserts were weighed to the nearest 0.01 mg, whereas the greater mass of the alumina inserts required a higher range on the balance, allowing their weight measurements to be determined only to the nearest 0.1 mg.

Throughout wear exposure, all inserts were removed from their chambers, cleaned, and weighed as described above approximately every 5.7×10^5 cycles.

Wear weight loss was converted to volumetric loss by dividing by the density reported in the material certifications. Volumetric loss was plotted as a function of cycles and least squares linear regression was used to determine a slope (representative of the wear rate) from zero to 5×10^6 cycles.

No attempt was made to determine the progressive weight loss of the ceramic femoral bearings since it was anticipated that a significant amount of metal transfer would occur from the Ti6Al4V trunnion fixtures, severely compromising the meaning of any measurement. In fact, unpublished efforts to remove metal transfer using an aggressive media introduces a significant alumina weight loss artifact, sometimes exceeding the amount of actual wear.

Other experimental techniques typically employed in examining gravimetric wear among different polyethylenes, such as the use of fatigue/soak controls, were not exercised in this study. The experience in this laboratory suggests that these effects influence the polyethylene wear rate by < 2% at 5×10^6 cycles, clearly insufficient to effect the conclusion drawn upon comparing the CoCr:UHMWPE couple to alumina:alumina.

Results

The overall weight loss average at 5×10^6 cycles was 0.3 mg (s.d. = 0.1 mg) and 166.06 mg (s.d. = 13.47 mg) for alumina and polyethylene inserts, respectively. This represents a 600X increase in the mass of debris released from polyethylene inserts compared to alumina. Using density values

Table 1 Gravimetric Wear Results for Acetabular Inserts

CoCr:UHMWPE		
Spec. No.	Insert Weight Loss at 5 x 10⁶ Cycles	Volumetric Wear Rate*
17451	186.05 mg	38.54 mm³/10⁶ cycles
17452	160.74 mg	32.74 mm³/10⁶ cycles
17453	160.80 mg	33.68 mm³/10⁶ cycles
17454	156.64 mg	31.71 mm³/10⁶ cycles
mean:	166.06 mg	34.17 mm³/10⁶ cycles
std. dev.:	13.47 mg	3.02 mm³/10⁶ cycles
Alumina:Alumina		
Spec. No.	Insert Weight Loss at 5 x 10⁶ Cycles**	(See Note #)
17210	0.3 (0.1) mg	
17211	0.4 (0.1) mg	
17212	0.4 (0.1) mg	
17213	0.1 (0.1) mg	
mean:	0.3 mg	
std. dev.:	0.1 mg	

* The convention for reporting polyethylene wear rate under hip joint simulation is the slope of the wear volume vs. cycles curve determined using least squares linear regression.

** Since no progressive weight loss was demonstrated after the first weighing, the listed value represents an average for the nine subsequent weighing intervals. The standard deviation is in parentheses.

\# Since linear correlation is poor (r ≈ 0.5) and an early wear-in period is demonstrated, a wear *rate* through 5 x 10⁶ cycles is misleading.

provided in material certifications, 3.980 g/cm³ for alumina and 0.937 g/cm³ for polyethylene, the difference in the volume of debris produced is 2000X. Given that the biological response to debris is less likely to be influenced by mass, the volumetric comparison (which is more readily related to number of particles, surface area, etc.) provides a more appropriate portrayal of relative burden. Scientific use of significant digits prevents more precise representation of relative wear.

Individual wear couple results are listed in Table 1. Figure 3 provides graphical representation of the average wear volume versus cycles.

The average volumetric wear rate exhibited by the polyethylene inserts, determined using least squares linear regression, was 34.17 mm³/10⁶ cycles (s.d. = 3.02 mm³/10⁶ cycles). As discussed in greater detail below, it became inappropriate to assign a wear rate for alumina inserts since the linear correlation coefficient was poor, averaging approximately 0.56.

SEM Observations

Non-worn surfaces are predominantly featureless, with occasional pores and residual polishing marks. After extensive scanning, the only evidence of wear encountered on worn femoral bearings appeared as grain relief, projected to be associated with preferential polishing of crystallo-

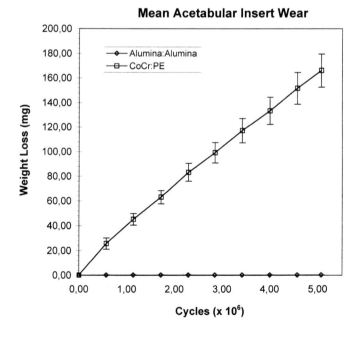

Fig. 3 Wear volume vs. cycles curves based on gravimetric measurements and material densities. Error bars represent ± one standard deviation.

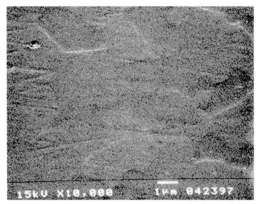

Fig. 4 SEM photomicrograph of worn alumina bearing surface after 5×10^6 cycles of hip joint simulation. Mag. 10,000X

graphic planes on the articulating surface, see Figure 4. This surface wear feature appears to be submicron in depth.

Discussion

Accuracy of Wear Measurement and Alumina Wear-in Period

The reproducibility of the scale was reported and confirmed to be 0.1 mg in the higher range necessary to weigh the alumina components. Assuming a normal distribution, approximately 95% of readings taken on a constant mass are expected to lie within ± 0.2 mg about the true mean. As shown in the apparent weight loss vs. cycles curves for the alumina components, Figure 5, the data scatter beyond the first weighing interval clearly fall within the expected error of the scale. ASTM E 178 (4) criteria was employed in determining whether the time zero average weight was an outlier and, if so, whether the apparent weight loss exhibited during the first 570K cycles was real or due to scale limitations. This exercise revealed that the subtle increase at the start of the test was indeed real at the 95% confidence level, indicating that the ceramic components had undergone a wear-in period within the first 570K cycles, producing an average 0.3 mg weight loss. This corresponds to a debris volume of 0.1 mm^3. To provide some perspective, this wear volume is approximately equivalent to that of two 450 μm diameter beads used in producing porous coatings on orthopaedic implants.

Since the variability in apparent wear produced by the four ceramic couples exceeds the reproducibility of the *less* accurate range on the scale, employment of a more accurate balance (i.e., that which provides a 0.01 mg standard deviation about the average weight of ceramic components)

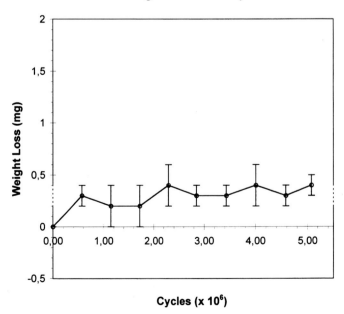

Fig. 5 Average wear mass vs. cycles for alumina inserts (n = 4). Error bars represent ± one standard deviation at each weighing interval. The shaded area depicts ± one standard deviation of the mean weight loss throughout 5×10^6 cycles (which is also equal to the standard deviation of the scale, or 0.1 mg) and is located about the overall mean weight loss, 0.3 mg.

would provide little benefit. Hence, gravimetric assessment of wear is likely to be unsuitable for comparing the extremely low wear rates among ceramic couples.

Comparison to Published Results for Ceramic:Ceramic

Previous researchers have clearly demonstrated an *in-vitro* reduction in wear of Al_2O_3:Al_2O_3 versus metal:PE – typically one or two orders of magnitude (5, 6). Overall, the reported clinical wear rates appear to exceed the expectations based on previous *in-vitro* joint simulation data, with the degree of *in-vivo* wear reduction ranging two or three orders of magnitude (7, 8, 9). The wear laboratory results presented herein, obtained using contemporary joint simulation model and technique, are consistent with reported *in-vivo* wear levels.

In addition to the material improvements, the lower wear rate compared to other *in-vitro* studies may also be a result of a superiorly located and 0° oriented acetabular specimen employed in this study, which avoids the mortar-and-pestle effect and containment of debris created by testing with the cup positioned below the femoral bearing. The use of „anatomic" in describing cup orientation has been oversimplified. Although a superior cup is anatomically relevant, its horizontal 0' orientation is not. Since the *in-vivo* cup inclination is believed to affect the clinical performance of ceramic couples, future *in-vitro* studies should consider an anatomically-relevant inclined acetabular specimen orientation.

The manifestation of wear in the form of grain relief on the femoral bearing surface is identical to that published by Boutin (7) for clinically-retrieved devices, corroborating the similarity in relative wear reduction.

Although intentionally not pursued in this study, the lack of explanation of whether literature reported wear rates are determined from measuring *both* articulating components comprising the hard:hard bearing couple is disquieting. In studying polyethylene wear, we can disregard the contribution of the much harder femoral bearing; however, in hard:hard bearing couples, the debris arising from the femoral bearing component becomes significant. At 60° cup inclination, the ratio of insert:bearing wear rate is approximately 3.3:1 according to Walter (10). At 45°, this ratio decrease to 2:1. This study, in effect, models a horizontal cup orientation (0° inclination). In regards to the effect of bearing wear on the overall debris generation, a conservative approach may be to assume a 1:1 ratio of insert:bearing wear, thereby doubling the calculated debris burden.

Comparison to Published Results for Metal:Metal

The amount of debris produced by the ceramic couples tested herein is approximately one order of magnitude less than that reported for contemporary metal:metal couples under in-vitro hip joint simulation (11, 12, 13). A volumetric comparison of debris generation would approximately double the reduction in wear in comparing ceramic:ceramic to metal:metal. In-vitro metal:metal wear also appears to exhibit a run-in period early in testing.

Conclusions

1. The average wear exhibited by 28 mm alumina acetabular inserts positioned superiorly under hip joint simulation is 0.3 mg (s.d. = 0.1 mg) at 5×10^6 cycles, representing a 0.1 mm^3 wear volume. The generation of this debris occurs during a wear-in period within the first 570K cycles of testing. This value excludes the contribution of alumina bearings which represent an additional source of debris.
2. The average wear volume of 28 mm UHMWPE inserts tested concurrently is approximately 2000X that of the alumina inserts, based on a 600X greater weight loss at 5×10^6 cycles.
3. The wear of alumina components under ideal sliding conditions appears as occasional grain relief observable under SEM examination at 10,000X magnification. At 5×10^6 cycles of hip joint simulation, the depth of material removal was less than approximately 0.2 µm.
4. Compared to literature values, the mass of debris generated by the ceramic:ceramic couple is approximately an order of magnitude less than that reported for *in-vitro* metal:metal articulation.

References

1 ASTM F 648 „Ultra-High Molecular Weight Polyethylene Powder and Fabricated Form for Surgical Implants"

2 Paul, J.P., „Forces Transmitted by Joints in the Human Body, Lubrication and Wear in Living and Artificial Human Joints," Proc. Inst. Mech., Eng., 181 (3J), 8–15, 1966/67.
3 Liao, Y.S., Benya, P.D., McKellop, H., „Stability of Serum as a Lubricant in Wear Simulator Tests of Prosthetic Joints," Trans. Fifth World Biomaterials Congress, 871, 1996.
4 ASTM E 178 „Standard Practice for Dealing with Outlying Observations," Vol. 14.02, American Society for Testing and Materials, Philadelphia, 1996.
5 Semlitsch, M., Lehmann, M., Weber, H., Doerre, E., Willert, H.G., „New Prospects for a Prolonged Functional Life-Span of Artificial Hip Joints by Using the Material Combination Polyethylene / Aluminum Oxide Ceramic / Metal," J. Biomed. Mater. Res., 11:537–52, 1977.
6 Wallbridge, J., Dowson, D., Roberts, E.W., „The Wear Characteristics of Sliding Pairs of High Density Polycrystalline Aluminum Oxide under both Dry and Wet Conditions," in Luderna, K.C. (ed.): Wear of Materials, New York, Amer. Soc. of Mech. Eng., 202–11, 1983.
7 Boutin, P., Christel, P., Dorlot, J.M., Meunier, A., de Roquancourt, A., Blanquaert, D., Herman, S., Sedel, L., Witvoet, J., „The Use of Dense Alumina-Alumina Ceramic Combination in Total Hip Replacement," J. Biomed. Mater. Res., 22, 1203–1232, 1988.
8 Clarke, I.C., Willman, G., „Structural Ceramics in Orthopedics," in Cameron, H.U. (ed.): Bone Implant Interface, St. Louis, Mosby, 203–52, 1994.
9 Doerre, E., „Ceramic Components for Hip Joint Prostheses: 18 Years of Experience," Trans. Fourth World Congress Biomaterials, Berlin, 17, 1992.
10 Walter, A., „On the Material and the Tribology of Alumina-Alumina Couplings for Hip Joint Prostheses," Clin. Ortho. Rel. Res., 282, 31–46, 1992.
11 Chan, F.W., Bobyn, J.D., Medley, J.B., Krygier, J.J., Yue, S., Tanzer, M., „Engineering Issues and War Performance of Metal on Metal Hip Implants," Clin. Ortho. Rel. Res., 333, 96–107, 1996.
12 Farrar, R., Schmidt, M.B., „The Effect of Diametral Mismatch on Wear Between head and Cup for Metal on Metal Articulations," Trans. 43rd Ann. Mtg. ORS, 71, 1997.
13 Scott, R.A., Schroeder, D.W., „The Effect of Radial Mismatch on the Wear of Metal on Metal Hip Prosthesis: A Hip Simulator Study," Trans. 43rd Ann. Mtg. ORS, 764, 1997.

3.4 Friction Induced Temperature Increase of Hip Implants

G. Bergmann, F. Graichen, A. Rohlmann

Introduction

Friction is much higher in artificial than in natural hip joints. It can therefore be assumed that hip implants warm up more. This effect will, among others, depend on the materials used for articulation components. It can be assumed that warming up is most severe during continuous activities accompanied by high hip contact forces as walking. The temperatures finally reached have never been measured in vivo. Goal of this study was to obtain realistic data allowing to judge whether friction induced peak temperatures can cause tissue damage or increase implant wear.

Methods

Clinically proven artificial hip joints were instrumented with three strain gauges inside the neck and inductively powered telemetry devices to allow wireless measurement of the hip contact forces in vivo (1). Two models were fabricated, both with titanium stems, ceramic heads (Biolox forte) and polyethylene cups.

The first model (9) was cemented, had one four-channel telemetry device and only one temperature sensor (sensor Ta) in the middle of the implant neck (Fig. 1, implant type I). Originally this sensor was aimed at compensating the temperature drift of the electronics. This endoprosthesis was implanted in five joints of four patients for up to nine years and a variety of activities was investigated (1 to 8). By chance remarkable temperature increases were found during walking in patient EB who got instrumented implants on both sides. This observation raised the question whether the final temperatures can cause tissue damage or increase polyethylene wear.

To investigate this problem a second kind of hip implant was developed (10). It is hollow inside stem and neck (Fig. 2, implant type II). Stem and socket are fixed without cement. Additionally to

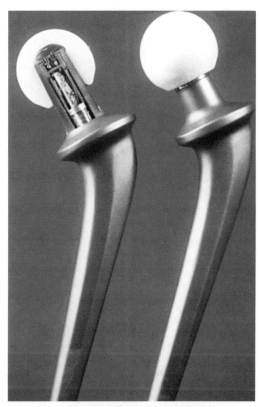

Fig. 1 Instrumented hip joint implant (type I). Measurement of hip contact force and one temperature Ta inside the neck. One four-channel telemetry with integrated coil for inductive power supply transmits the signals.

the three strain gauges in the neck, used for measuring the hip contact forces, is has eight temperature sensors (T1 to T8) distributed along the whole length of neck and stem (Fig. 6). Two eight-channel telemetries with one additional temperature sensor each (Ta and Tb) are employed. This endoprosthesis was used in five joints of four patients. The patient with two instrumented im-

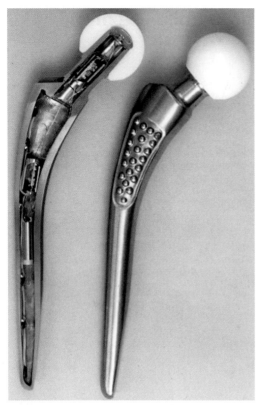

Fig. 2 Instrumented hip joint implant (type II) Measurement of hip contact force, 8 temperatures along neck and shaft (T1 to T8), and the temperatures at the locations of the two telemetries (Ta and Tb). A separate internal coil powers both eight-channel telemetries. Sensor locations see Fig. 6.

plants got, as all others, a polyethylene cup on the right side (KWR) but a ceramic (Biolox forte) cup on the left side (KWL).

For measuring the joint temperatures the patients first rest to achieve nearly steady state temperature conditions. Then they walk in a gymnasium at a speed of 3–4 km/h until warming up of the implant is finished and rest again to observe cooling down. Hip contact forces and temperature signals are both displayed real time on a computer monitor and recorded on video tape together with the images. These measurements can only be taken later than about one year after surgery when the patients walk normal again and can do this for about one hour.

Results

Until now measurements were taken in three patients. From patient EB (body weight BW = 640 N) data were obtained from the left and right hip joint (EBL and EBR, Fig. 3). His rectal body temperature was additionally recorded. Complete data were obtained from the right joint of patient KWR (BW = 720 N, Fig. 4 and 5). For patient HSR only preliminary measurements 2 months after implantation could be obtained until now (BW = 820 N, Fig. 6).

It takes about one hour for the implant temperatures to reach their final steady state values (Fig. 3 and 4). In EBR a maximum of 40.6°C was found at sensor Ta (Fig. 3) which is located on the upper telemetry circuit (Fig. 5). In EBL the highest value

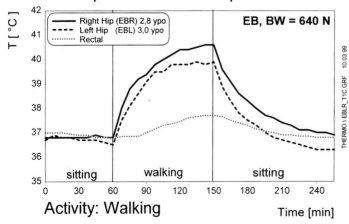

Fig. 3 Temperature changes during walking and resting. Patient EB, left (EBL) and right (EBR) hip joint, 2.8–3 years postoperatively. Shown are the temperatures Ta of the upper telemetry and the rectal body temperature. Implant type I.

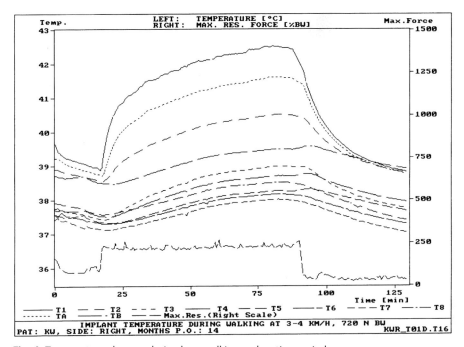

Fig. 4 Temperature changes during long walking and resting periods
Patient KWR, right hip joint, 14 months postoperatively. Shown are 9 temperatures along the whole length of the implant (left scale in °C) plus the peak joint force (lowest curve with right scale in percent of body weight). Sensor locations see Fig. 5. Implant type II.

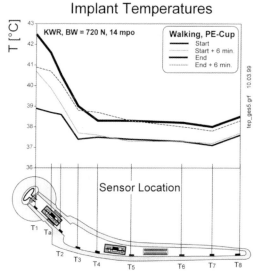

Fig. 5 Temperature changes during long walking and resting periods
Temperatures along the whole length of the implant at 4 different times: start of walking, after 6 minutes of walking, final values after walking and decrease after 6 minutes of resting. Data from Fig. 4.

of Ta was 39.9°C. In KWR up to 42.5°C was observed for T1 (Fig. 4). In these patients the peak joint forces during the stance phase of walking were about 270%BW (percent of body weight). The temperature distribution along the length of the implant of KWR, charted for 4 different instants of time (Fig. 5), shows that warming up during walking predominantly takes place at the implant head and neck. The shaft temperatures increase much less and nearly uniform along the whole stem length. This increase of the shaft is about the same as the increase of the rectal body temperature (Fig. 3). Highest temperatures are found at sensor T1 which is closest to the frictional interface between head and socket. From the difference between T1 and Ta in KWR (Fig. 4 and 5) it can be concluded that the final temperatures at T1 in EBL and EBR (Fig. 3), which could not be measured, were about 1° higher than the values displayed for Ta.

Frictional heating let the implant warm up nearly immediately (Fig. 3 and 4). The temperature increase at the beginning of walking is very steep. Resting also causes very fast temperature

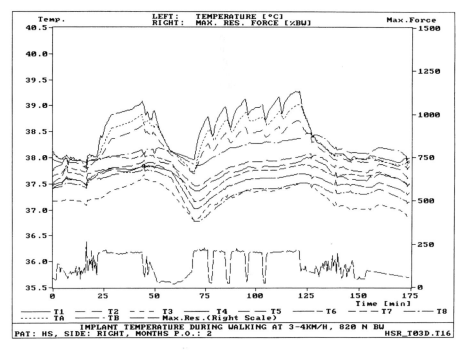

Fig. 6 Temperature changes during short walking and resting periods
Patient HSR, right hip joint, 2 months postoperatively. Further explanations see Fig. 4.

changes. Half of the total temperature in- and decrease is reached after only 6 minutes (Fig. 5).

The early postoperative data from HSR contain short periods of walking with intermediate rests (Fig. 6). A similar temperature behaviour as in the other patients can be observed. However, a detailed analysis shows that the increase during the first minutes of walking is more than two times lower than in EBL, EBR and KWR (Fig. 3 and 4). Is can therefore be assumed that the final temperatures after walking for an hour will be much lower in this patient, too.

Discussion

Temperatures directly at the frictional interface between head and ball could not be measured with the instrumented hip implants. Those temperatures and the heat distribution in the biological tissue surrounding the implant will be calculated in the future using a finite element model. This model will be tuned to simulate the real conditions found in the patients. It can then be employed to simulate other material combinations than those used in this study. It will also answer the question whether or not the temperatures in bone and joint capsule are high enough to cause biological damage and contribute to implant loosening.

Even without such finite element calculations it is certain, however, that friction temperature at the cup and ball surface is much higher than the values measured at sensor T1 which is closest to the head surface. Interface values of much more than 50°C can be assumed for the investigated material combination of ceramic head and polyethylene cup. Certainly polyethylene wear is then much higher than at a body temperature of 37°C. Future simulator wear tests should consider this.

The dependency of implant temperatures from the material combination of head and cup will be investigated in patient KW. These measurements will show whether a ceramic cup helps to reduce the implant temperature. Furthermore measurements during cycling will be performed in several patients. This activity reduces the hip force magnitudes to only about 25% of those during walking for comparable power consumption of the patient. Such intraindividual data will reveal which role the force magnitudes play for the final implant temperatures and how much warming up of the muscles contributes to the thermal effects.

The preliminary data from HSR indicate much lower temperatures in this patient than in EBL, EBR and KW, although the peak joint forces were comparable in all cases. Besides the joint force magnitudes still unknown other factors probably play a role in the frictional temperature behaviour of hip implants. One factor could be that heat dissipation depends on the individually different circulatory system of the patients.

The fast response of the temperatures to both loading situations, walking and resting, probably makes it impractical to keep the final implant temperatures limited by intermittent rests when walking long distances. Otherwise walking and resting periods had both to be as short as 5 or 6 minutes.

Acknowledgement

This work was supported by the German Research Society. We thank all patients for their cooperation.

References

1. Bergmann G, Graichen F, Siraky J, Jendrzynski H, Rohlmann A (1988) Multichannel Strain Gauge Telemetry for Orthopaedic Implants. J. Biomech. 21: 169–176
2. Bergmann G, Graichen F, Rohlmann A (1993) Hip joint forces during walking and running, measured in two patients. J. Biomech. 26: 969–990
3. Bergmann G, Correa da Silva M, Neff G, Rohlmann A, Graichen F (1994) Evaluation of ischial weight bearing orthoses, based on in vivo hip joint force measurements. Clin. Biomechanics 9: 225–234
4. Bergmann G, Graichen F, Rohlmann A (1995) Is Staircase Walking a Risk for the Fixation of Hip Implants? J. Biomech. 28: 535–553
5. Bergmann G, Kniggendorf H, Graichen F, Rohlmann A (1995) Influence of shoes and heel strike on the loading of hip implants. J. Biomech. 28: 817–827
6. Bergmann G (1997) In vivo Messung der Belastung von Hüftimplantaten. Dr. Köster, Berlin, ISBN 3-89574-233-3
7. Bergmann G, Graichen F, Rohlmann A (1997) Hip Joint Forces During Load Carrying. Clin. Orthop. Rel. Res. 335: 190–201
8. Bergmann G, Graichen F, Rohlmann A (1998) Loads acting at the hip joint. In: Sedel L, Cabanela ME (eds) Hip surgery – materials and developments. M. Dunitz, London 1–8
9. Graichen F, Bergmann G (1991) Four-channel telemetry system for in vivo measurement of hip joint forces. J. Biomed. Eng. 13: 370–374
10. Graichen F, Bergmann G, Rohlmann A (submitted) Hip endoprosthesis for in vivo measurement of joint forces and temperature. J. Biomechanics

3.5 Wear study in the Alumina-zirconia System

C. Kaddick, H.G. Pfaff

Abstract

Alumina/alumina couplings proved to sufficiently reduce wear in total hip arthroplasty. The increasing requirements of THR causes ongoing researches for new ceramic materials and combinations. One of the potential solutions are mixtures between alumina and zirconia ceramics resulting in new materials with different mechanical strength and wear resistance than the pure components.

The aim of the herein presented study was to test various combinations between alumina and zirconia ceramics using a screening test according to ISO 6474 (ring-on-disc). A total of 10 different combinations (3 specimens each) has been tested under demineralized water and the wear volume as well as the surface parameters have been determined. Alumina/alumina couplings served as a reference.

The results presented herein clearly demonstrate the influence of the zirconia content on the tribologic behavior using the ring-on-disc method. High amounts of zirconia at both sides (ring and disc) lead to catastrophic failure (up to 45 mm^3 wear volume). Best results have been achieved for the alumina/alumina coupling already in clinical use as well as for couplings with small amounts of zirconia (0.008 mm^3 wear volume).

Introduction

Osteolysis induced by PE wear particles is considered to be one of the key problems in hip arthroplasty. In the last decade a large research effort has been undertaken to improve the wear behavior of hip joints by the introduction of alternative bearing materials. Alumina on alumina as well as metal on metal hard bearings are now clinically introduced and represent the new generation of alternate bearings. In the last decade ultra high molecular weight polyethylene underwent two iterations of technical improvement with cross-linked PE now being introduced. With the improvement of the longevity younger and more active patients can receive a THR. Therefor the requirements to prosthesis increase steadily. In the following study the wear performance of new ceramic materials having improved mechanical properties is investigated. Basic wear mechanisms and wear modes of ceramic materials are highlighted and compared to other materials.

1. Wear behavior of ceramic on ceramic bearings

The wear couple of endoprosthesis represents a complex tribological system which is subject to a variety of influence parameters. Material properties, surface properties, interactions between the wear couple, lubricant, chemical influences, change of material properties during service time and chemical interactions influence the wear behavior. To describe the behavior of a tribological system a model with three different wear modes is used [15, 13] (s. Fig. 1).

In mode one the system reveals very low wear rates. If the main influence parameter (e. g. time, force, chemistry) increases, the wear rates increase exponentially and the wear mechanisms change. Mode 3 is characterized by a steady state

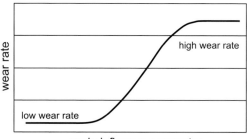

Fig. 1 Transition between low and high wear rate

Table 1 Wear mechanisms of wear couplings in THR

Wear Coupling	wear mechanism			critical parameter	Reference
	mode 1	mode 2	mode 3		
Me/UHMWPE	grooving wear	material degradation		surface roughness, wear distance, material stability	[8, 2, 10, 4]
Ce/UHMWPE	grooving wear	material degradation		surface roughness, wear distance, material stability	[8, 2, 10, 4]
ME/ME	grooving wear		material transfer	contact pressure, 3rd particles, surface roughness	[14]
Ce/Ce	particle erosion, mild abrasion	particle erosion, 3rd body wear	3rd body wear	contact pressure, 3rd particles	[16, 12]

wear rate on a high level and different wear mechanisms compared to mode 1. Wear couples to be used in THR are to operate in a steady state type 1 wear mode.

In the wearing process surface is usually destroyed. On the other hand, functional surface can be generated (s. Fig. 2). If the portion of the surface area destroyed by wear is equal or smaller than the new generated surface, the wear couple runs in a stable type 1 mode. If the share of the surface area generated by wear is larger than the newly formed functional area the functional area decreases and the wear rate increases continuously. Operating in this type 2 mode a wear couple reveals a limited service time and changes into wear mode type 3 where completely destroyed functional surface areas articulate against each other and the wear rates are extremely high.

The wear behavior of nowadays alumina ceramic bearings can be characterized by two mechanisms. A very limited amount of grain pull out is observed and as well areas showing mild abrasion wear phenomena [12, 16]. The alumina ceramic bearings operate in a steady state wear rate mode type 1. A transition into mode 2 or even mode 3 can only be induced by third particle wear if the particles exceed a critical particle size and quantity. In developmental zirconia on zirconia coupling this process is initiated by the phase transformation of the Y-TZP material [5, 9].

Regarding other material systems which are used in THR different wear phenomena can be observed. The main wear mechanisms and critical parameters of wear systems commonly used in THR are shown in the table 2. Hard and hard bearing systems can be well characterized by the three

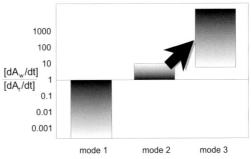

Fig. 2 Wear modes of hard on hard bearings (mode 1: steady state wear, low wear rate, particle erosion compensated by mild abrasion; mode 2: functional surface being reduced continuously, 3rd body wear induced by wear debris; mode 3: no functional surface, worn surfaces articulating against each other). A_w non functional surface generated by wear, A_f newly formed functional surface

mode wear model as a digital wear behavior. Ceramic systems show a pronounced mode 3 behavior. Metal on metal systems can not be described with that model, but the critical wear parameters are very well studied. Systems with a polyethylene articulation show a different behavior. Hard on PE bearings operate in a type 1 mode wear mode at a higher wear rate. The critical parameters are surface roughness of the hard counterface and the long term stability of the PE [2, 8, 4].

The purpose of the herein presented study was to detect the wear behavior of various ceramic couplings corresponding to the defined classifications (mode 1 to mode 3). According to the princi-

Table 2 Properties of the investigated materials

Material		100-Alumina	75-Alumina	20-Alumina	Y-TZP
Alumina content	%	> 99,7	75	20	0
[Zirconia + Yttria] content	%	0	24	80	100
Bending strength	MPa	550	1100	900	900
Hardness	HV05	2200	1800	1400	1200
K_{1C}	MPa m$^{1/2}$	4	10	n.m.	9

ples of screening tests at all, mode 3 couplings can be excluded from further evaluations.

2. Materials and methods

Alumina and Zirconia are both materials used in hip arthroplasty. Alumina shows a very high hardness, wear resistance and an extreme chemical stability. Alumina is present in the stable crystalline alpha-phase. Y-TZP ceramics are characterized by high strength. But as the tetragonal zirconia represents the stabilized high temperature modification, it is always susceptible to phase transformation, which is associated with a degradation of the mechanical properties [11, 3]. The combination of the positive properties of alumina and zirconia seems to be desirable for a ceramic bearing material. For that reason the system alumina-zirconia was investigated. Specimen out of four materials i. e. alumina, Y-TZP and two alloys of zirconia and alumina were manufactured. Characteristic properties of these materials are listed in table 1.

The alumina material is a hot isostatically pressed type alumina (BIOLOX *forte*). The 20-alumina is a hot isostatically pressed Y-TZP with 20 w% alumina in the matrix, to harden the zirconia. The 75-alumina is a hot isostatically pressed zirconia toughened alumina. Zirconia particles are homogeneously dispersed in the alumina matrix to improve strength and toughness. The investigated zirconia is a hot isostatically pressed Y-TZP material.

A total of 30 couplings has been tested using the ring-on-disc method according to ISO 6474. A flat ring is pressed against a flat plate with a constant force and articulated in reciprocating manner. The surface pressure is set to 9.37 MPa. The test runs at 1 Hz frequency and is stopped after 100 hours resulting in a total number of cycles of n = 960 000. All tests have been performed in demineralized water. To avoid high temperatures caused by friction [5], external cooling to 20°C has been used.

The quality of the surface has been determined by five measurements prior and after the test (according to ISO 4287-1) using a roughness measuring system (Mitutoyo 178-885D, Mitutoyo). In addition to the conventional parameter Ra, Ry and Rt the values for peaks and flutes at the surface have been determined using the parameter Rpk and Rvk (cut off = 0.08 µm).

To evaluate the wear volume, surface measurements of the wear track are performed at six equally distributed points (s. Fig. 3). A custom made software (EndoLab GmbH) calculated the resulting wear volume.

Alumina and Zirconia ceramic has been tested in varying combinations and compositions.

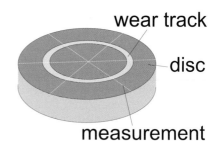

Fig. 3 Measurement of the wear track to determine the wear volume at six points.

Table 3 Composition of the specimens tested (each group n = 3).

Coupling No.	alumina/zirconia ring [%] / [%]	alumina/zirconia disc [%] / [%]
1	100 / 0	100 / 0
2	100 / 0	75 / 24
3	100 / 0	20 / 80
4	100 / 0	0 / 100
5	75 / 24	75 / 24
6	20 / 80	75 / 24
7	20 / 80	20 / 80
8	0 / 100	75 / 24
9	0 / 100	20 / 80
10	0 / 100	0 / 100

3. Results

The initial roughness parameters (Ra, Ry and Rt) showed normal values of polished ceramic surfaces. According to the wear volume detected after the test, the change of the surface varied from „improved" to „catastrophic". Two examples of this behavior are shown in Fig. 4 and 5.

The total amount of wear volume differed from 0.008 mm³ (coupling 6) to 45.414 mm³ (coupling 9). To enable comparison between the different types of compositions, a three dimensional plot as shown in Fig. 6 has been generated. Each dot plotted represents the mean value of n = 3 tests.

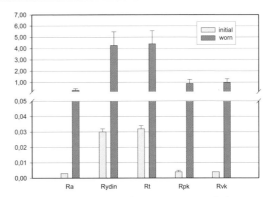

Fig. 5 Coupling 9: Surface parameter of the ring before and after the test showing catastrophic failure.

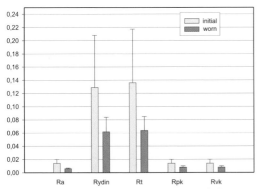

Fig. 4 Coupling 2: Surface parameter of the ring before and after the test showing improvement of the surface due to run-in period.

4. Discussion

The results presented herein clearly demonstrate the influence of the zirconia content on the tribologic behavior using the ring-on-disc method. High amounts of zirconia at both sides (ring and disc) lead to catastrophic failure. Best results have been achieved for the alumina/alumina coupling already in clinical use as well as for couplings with small amounts of zirconia.

It can be stated that wear volumes above 0.1 mm³ correspond to wear mode 3 of ceramic/ceramic couplings. The results confirm the „digital" wear behavior of ceramic couplings. This

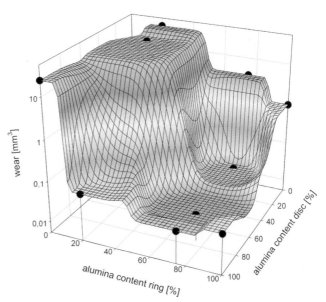

Fig. 6 Wear volume of different combinations of alumina and zirconia couplings. The difference to 100% represents the zirconia content.

again addresses the fact that small changes of the composition or of the in service condition may lead to large effects in-vivo.

Due to the fact that the test setup described by ISO 6474 has to be regarded as a screening test there are some limitations transferring the data obtained herein to medical components:

First of all is the increase of temperature observed: Limiting the maximum temperature by external cooling proved to be a sufficient tool prevent loosening of the specimens from the specimen holder. This fact may be satisfying for the laboratory staff but some questions may arise: Zirconia is well known for thermal instability leading to roughening of the surface. Decreasing the temperature of the surrounding test fluid will not prevent the specimen from heating up at the microscopic level of the surfaces in contact. The onset of phase transition can not be excluded. Again this raises the question whether this important failure mechanism will occur in-vivo. Recent investigations [1, 7] show that there is an increase of temperature in-vivo. The lack of data for the temperature of the heat source itself prevents final conclusions.

The contact conditions of the test itself differ from clinical applications in use. Due to the flat on flat geometry, peak stresses occur at the edges of the contact zone. Those regions of high mechanical stresses may initiate local failure and subsequent macroscopic failure of the whole contact zone. This behavior may be enhanced by the hydrothermal effects described above.

Regarding the in-vivo situation, the locus of high stresses moves, whereas in the test set up described by ISO 6474, the locus does not move.

Both effects enhance the onset of mode 3 failure of ceramic couplings tested herein. In consequence, the results represent a worst-case scenario including a high safety factor.

5. Conclusion

The investigated wear couples show wear rates either at a low level or at a high level and confirm the digital wear behavior of ceramics. Wear couples generating high wear rates consist of at least one component with a high zirconia content. All the wear couplings with a low wear rate consist of materials with a high alumina content. The influence of the zirconia contents on the wear performance can be clearly shown. As long as either one wear partner consists of 100% zirconia or both wear partners have a dominant share of zirconia in the matrix the investigated wear couples operate at a high wear rate in wear mode type 3. As long as pure alumina articulates against pure alumina or at least one alumina wear component articulates against an alumina containing wear partner low wear rates in wear mode 1 can be observed. Therefore it may be concluded that wear couples on the high alumina side of the system zirconia – alumina will represent wear systems with excellent wear properties and excellent material properties. Taking into account that with the decreasing age of the patients receiving a hip joint long term stability and high mechanical strength are prerequisites for a successful use in hip arthroplasty further investigations of this material system may reveal new ceramic bearings.

Material combinations with high zirconia contents seem to be associated with a higher risk of failure in a wear application, which is introduced to enhance the longevity of a hip joint prosthesis.

Literature

1 *Bergmann G*: Loading and friction induced temperature increase of hip implants. Realiability and long term results of ceramics in orthopaedics. in: ed. Sedel, Willmann. Enke, 1999
2 *Besong AA, Hailey JL, Ingham E, Stone M, Wroblewski BM, Fisher F*: A study of the combined effects of shelf ageing following irridation in air and counterface roughness on the wear of UHMWPE. Biomed Mater Eng 7 (1997) 59–65.
3 *Chevalier J, Drouin JM, Cales B*: Temperature aging behavior of zirconia hip joint heads, in: Sedel L (ed.) Bioceramics 10. Pergamon., Elsevier Sci. Ltd., Oxford, 1997, p.135–138.
4 *Davidson JA.*: Characteristics of metal and ceramic total hip bearing surfaces and their effect on long-term ultra high molecular weight polyethylene wear. Clin Orthop Rel Res 294 (1993) 361–378
5 *Früh HJ, Willmann G, Pfaff HG*: Wear characteristics of ceramic-on-ceramic for hip endoprostheses. Biomat 18 (1997) 873–876.
6 ISO 6474, Implants for surgery: ceramic materials based on high purity alumina. 2nd edn, 1994
7 *Lu Z, McKellop H*: Frictional heating of bearing materials tested in a hip joint wear simulator. Proc Instn Mech Engrs 211(1997)101–108
8 *McKellop HA*: Wear modes, mechanisms, damage, and debris. Separating cause from effect in the wear of total hip replacements in: Total hip revision surgery. Galante et al (ed), Raven press, Ltd., New York 1995.
9 *Piconi C, Maccauro G*: Zirconia as a ceramic biomaterial. Biomat 20(1999)1–25

10 *Plitz W, Walter A*: Tribological aspects of metal/polymer couplings: in Buchhorn GH, Willert HG ed, Technical principals design and safety, 1994, Hofrege & Huber, Seattle
11 *Richter HG, Burger W, Osthues F*: Zirconia for medical implants – the role of strength properties. in: Andersson et al Bioceramics 7.Butterworth 1994.
12 *Saikko V, Pfaff HG*: Low wear and friction in alumina/alumina total hip joints. Acta Orthop Scan 69 (1998) 443–448.
13 *Schneider J*: Tribologisches Verhalten HfO2-laserlegierter Al_2O_3-Keramiken unter ungeschmierter Gleitbeanspruchung. IKM 018, Institut für Keramik im Maschinenbau, Universität Karlsruhe.
14 *Semlitsch M, Streicher RM, Weber H*: Verschleißraten von Pfannen und Kugeln aus CoCrMo-Gußlegierungen bei langzeitig implantierten Ganzmetall-Hüftprothesen. Orthopäde 18 (1989) 377–381
15 *Uetz H*: Abrasion und Erosion-Grundlagen und Betriebliche Erfahrungen Verminderungen. Hanser, München.
16 *Walter A*: On the material and the tribology of alumina-alumina couplings for hip joint prostheses. Clin Orthop 282 (1992) 31

3.6 Die Materialpaarung Zirkonoxid/Aluminiumoxid im Hüftgelenk – Eine Fallstudie
The Wear Couple Zirconia/Alumina in THR: A Case Study

M.M. Morlock, R. Nassutt, M. Honl, R. Janßen, G. Willmann

Abstract

A patient had complained about a squeaking noise in his total hip replacement, which ultimately required a revision surgery. The retrieved components were a ceramic cup and a ceramic femoral head which were in-vivo for 37 months. The analysis of these retrievals yielded the following results:

i. The acetabular component was a cementless fixed, monolithic cup made of alumina ceramics of the 1st generation (FRIALIT).
ii. The 32 mm femoral head was made of zirconia ceramics. The manufacturer is unknown.
iii. The linear wear of the socket was about 12 μm, the one of the head about 9 μm, i.e. the total wear rate was about 7 μm per year.
iv. Based on the evaluation of the articulating surface of the cup it must be concluded that the cup is not according to today's specification.

Concluding remarks

i. For satisfactory lubrication, a gap between the articulating surfaces is required. The observed high wear rate was either caused by a gap too small and/or by the unsatisfactory sphericity of the articulating surfaces. The resulting high stress concentrations in the ceramics caused detoriation of the microstructure, wear, possibly chipping, and 3 body wear.
ii. The combination of this retrieved wear couple was never approved. In order to prevent such problems, components of different producers should never be mixed and matched unless stated otherwise.
iii. Up to now there is no clinical experience with the wear couple zirconia ceramics-on-alumina ceramics. Therefore this couple should not be used clinically.

Einleitung

Die Gleitpaarung Aluminiumoxidkeramik/Aluminiumoxidkeramik für die Hüftendoprothetik ist unter tribologischen Gesichtspunkten die Kombination mit den geringsten Abrieb in-vitro und in-vivo (1, 2, 3, 4, 5). Somit bietet sie eine gute Option, die durch Partikel induzierte Osteolyse zu reduzieren (6, 7). Hierbei muß jedoch bedacht werden, daß Keramik nicht gleich Keramik ist. Auch wenn Aluminiumoxidkeramik und Zirkonoxidkeramik bzw. unterschiedliche Aluminumoxidkeramiken für den Laien schwer zu unterscheiden sind, so stellen die Zusammensetzung, das Gefüge und die Geometrie bzw. die Toleranzen der Keramik entscheidende Faktoren für die Abriebeigenschaften dar. Dies ist besonders bei der Zusammenstellung von Hart/Hartpaarungen zu beachten (8, 9, 10). Die vorliegende Fallstudie macht dies deutlich.

Anamnese

Ein 57-jähriger männlicher Patient wurde bei einer fortgeschrittenen Coxarthrose rechts (Abbildung 1a) mit einer zementfreien Hüft-TEP versorgt. Hierbei wurden ein zementfreier ABG Schaft (Howmedica, Kiel), eine Keramik-Schraubpfanne (Hersteller *FRIATEC, Mannheim – Friedrichsfeld*) und ein „neutraler" Keramikkopf (Hersteller unbekannt) kombiniert. 35 Monate postoperativ stellte sich der Patient erneut vor und beklagte ein Quietschgeräusch in der operierten Hüfte beim Treppensteigen bei ansonsten völlig schmerz- und problemfreien Befund. Die klinische Untersuchung ergab eine gute Beweglichkeit (Extension/Flexion 0–0–100), der röntgenologisch Befund zeigte keinerlei Anzeichen von Lockerung. Da das Geräuschphänomen nur in bestimmten Bewegungssituationen vom Patienten verursacht werden konnte, wurde zunächst eine intensive krankengymnastische Übungsbehand-

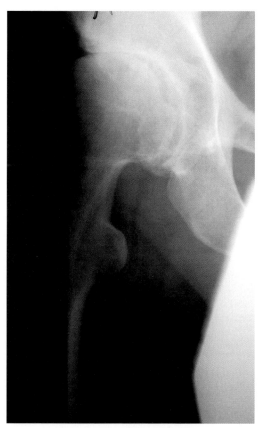 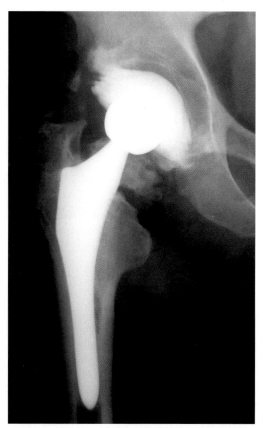

Abb. 1 Zustand (a) vor Erstoperation und (b) vor Revision.

lung für indiziert angesehen. 6 Monate später stellte sich der Patient erneut vor; die klinische und röntgenologische Untersuchungen (Abbildung 1b) ergaben den selben Befund wie zuvor. Da der Patient durch die zunehmenden Quietschgeräusche eine erhebliche Störung seiner Lebensqualität beklagte, entschloß man sich zur Wechseloperation, welche 2 Monate später durchgeführt wurde. Intraoperativ wurden keinerlei Lockerungsanzeigen festgestellt. Es wurde auf eine zementfrei implantierte Preß-Fit-Pfanne mit PE-Inlay und auf einen Keramikkopf aus Zirkoniumoxid gewechselt. Der Schaft wurde belassen. Der postoperative Verlauf gestaltete sich komplikationslos.

Methode

Die explantierte Pfanne und der Kopf wurden qualitativ und quantitativ analysiert. Mittels einer CNC-gesteuerten 3D-Koordinatenmeßmaschine (Mitutoyo BHN 305) wurden die Pfanne und der Kopf separat vermessen (Abbildung 2). Der Taster bestand aus einer Rubin-Kugel mit einem Durchmesser von 2 mm; die Meßgenauigkeit war ± 1μm. Mit einem Punkteraster von 0,2 mm wurde die Gleitfläche des Kopfes und der Pfanne in 13 Ebenen (jeweils durch den Pol des Prüfkörpers) abgetastet. Die so ermittelten ebenen Konturen wurden gespeichert und mittels eines Soll-Ist-Wert-Vergleiches zwischen Kugel- und Pfannenkontur wurden die Differenzen in den Abmessungen der korrespondierenden Gelenkpartner bestimmt. Für diesen Vergleich wurden zusätzlich mathematisch ideale Kreisgeometrien des Nenndurchmessers erzeugt, um isoliert Formabweichungen der einzelnen Bauteile zu ermitteln. Auffällige Oberflächenbereiche auf dem Kopf wurden zusätzlich mit einem tastenden Rauhigkeitsmeßsystem (Perthometer®) überprüft.

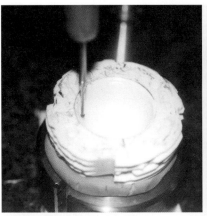 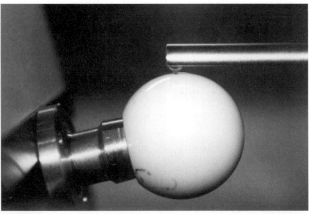

Abb. 2 Vermessung mit einem Rubinkugel-Taster auf der Mitutoyo BHN 305 (a) Aluminiumoxidkeramik – Schraubpfanne; (b) Zirkonoxidkeramik – Kopf.

Ergebnisse

Der Kopf und die Pfanne stammen von unterschiedlichen Herstellern und sind aus unterschiedlichen Materialien hergestellt. Der Kopf besteht aus einer Zirkonoxidkeramik (ZrO_2), die Pfanne aus Aluminiumoxidkeramik (Al_2O_3) der 1. Generation, d.h. einer Keramik gemäß ISO 6474 (1st ed. 1981) (11). Diese Norm wurde 1994 überarbeitet und verschärft (12). Man erkennt den Unterschied der Materialien bei Pfanne und Kopf gut auf dem Röntgenbild (Abbildung 1b): die Grenzlinie zwischen Pfanne und Kopf ist deutlich zu erkennen, was bei gleicher Keramik nicht der Fall wäre. Der Kopf aus Zirkonoxidkeramik erscheint als „absolut weiß", da Zirkonium (Zr) eine hohe Ordnungszahl besitzt und deswegen röntgenundurchlässiger als die Aluminiumoxidkeramik ist.

Die explantierte Pfanne ist eine monolithische, zementfrei zu implantierende Schraubpfanne aus Aluminiumoxidkeramik (Werkstoff FRIALIT der Fa. FRIATEC). Die Pfanne zeigt in ihrer äußeren Erscheinung teilweise beschädigte Gewindekanten mit Ausbrüchen. Der Kragen, bzw. die Kragenfläche weist bis in den Grenzbereich zur inneren polierten Gleitfläche Kratzspuren von metallischen Werkzeugen auf. Diese Spuren sind wahrscheinlich während der Revision entstanden. Die Gleitfläche selbst erscheint mit bloßem Auge unbeschädigt und auch nicht verfärbt. Eine zusätzliche Vermessung der randnahen Gleitfläche in Umfangsrichtung zeigt eine maximale Abweichung von der idealen Kugelgeometrie von etwa 8/100 mm (Abbildung 3), ein Wert, der weit über den

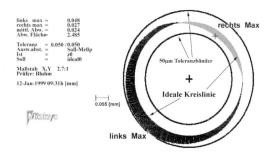

Abb. 3 Abweichungen der Pfanne von der idealen Kreisgeometrie auf der Gleitfläche im randnahen Bereich (Abweichung links Max: 48 µm, rechts Max: 27 µm).

heute üblichen Fertigungstoleranzen für Pfannen bzw. Pfanneneinsätze liegt.

Eine Betrachtung des Kopfes aus Zirkonoxidkeramik läßt eine Verfärbung in großen Bereichen erkennen. Die grundsätzliche Farbe des Kopfes ist weißlicher und weicht deutlich von der gelblichrötlichen der Pfanne ab. Eine Seite des Kopfes weist einen Bereich auf, der optisch matt wirkt und rauher ist als die restliche Oberfläche, ein sogenanntes Verschleißband. Dieser Bereich lag, der aus der Röntgendokumentation bekannten Lage (Schenkelhalswinkel) folgend, möglicherweise superior, also im Bereich der Hauptbelastungszone des Kopfes (Abbildung 4). Dieses Verschleißband ist auch bei der Konturvermessung deutlich wiederzuerkennen. Abbildung 5a zeigt einen Vergleich von Pfanne und Kopf, Abbildung 5b zusätzlich einen Vergleich der Kopfkontur mit einem mathematisch idealen Kreis. Der Vergleich mit

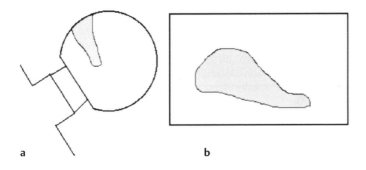

Abb. 4 (a) Schematische Darstellung des Hauptverschleißbandes auf dem Prothesenkopf und (b) auf der abgerollten Oberfläche.

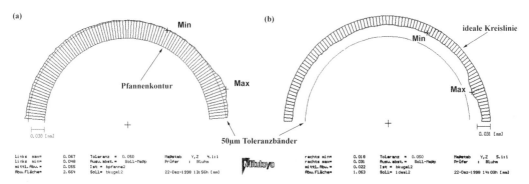

Abb. 5 (a) Ist/Soll Vergleich Pfanne und Kugel (Abweichungen Max: 67m, Min: 47 µm, Mittel: 55 µm); (b) Abweichung Kopfkontur von idealer Kugel (Max: 31 µm, Min: 18 µm, Mittel: 22 µm).

der Idealgeometrie macht deutlich, daß die Differenz hauptsächlich auf einen Oberflächendefekt auf dem Kopf zurückzuführen ist. Der Kopf ist in diesem Bereich deutlich verschlissen. Wenn man von einer ursprünglichen Passung von ca. 55 µm (⌀ Kopf um 55 µm kleiner als Innen-⌀ Pfanne) ausgeht, so ist die maximale Abweichung nach 3 Jahren in-situ ca. 12 µm (Ist/Soll Vergleich Pfanne-Kugel, Abbildung 5a), wovon ca. 9 µm dem Kopf zuzurechnen sind (Abweichung Kopfkontur von idealer Kugel, Abbildung 5b).

Diskussion

Künstliche Hüftgelenke sind komplexe Systeme, deren erfolgreiche Funktion von vielen Faktoren beeinflußt wird. Die hier untersuchte Pfanne weist für eine Hart/Hart-Paarung im Vergleich zu dem heutigen Standard deutliche zu hohe lokale Formabweichungen auf. Die Gleitfläche der Pfanne ist bis auf den Randbereich ansonsten jedoch praktisch nicht verschlissen. Der Kopf zeigt nach 3 Jahren Standzeit bereits deutliche Verschleißspuren. Er weist Oberflächenbereiche auf, die matt und rauh sind und als Vertiefungen von bis zu 9 µm charakterisiert werden können.

Auf der Basis langjähriger klinischer Erfahrung (13) besteht Konsens darüber, daß die Gleitpaarungen Aluminiumoxid/Polyethylen, Zirkonoxid/Polyethylen und Aluminiumoxid/Aluminiumoxid im Vergleich zu der am meisten gebräuchlichen Gleitpaarung Metall/Polyethylen die in-vivo Abriebrate deutlich reduzieren können (z.B. Sauer und Anthony) (14). Ebenso besteht Konsens darüber, daß die Gleitpaarung Zirkonoxid/Zirkonoxid nicht verwendet werden sollte (8). Bei der Gleitpaarung Zirkonoxid/Aluminiumoxid ist die Bewertung uneinheitlich: Früh et al. (9) haben auf der Basis von Ring-on-disk Versuchen geschlossen, daß diese Paarung ein hohes Risiko darstellt; Cales (15) dagegen berichtet von vielversprechenden Ergebnissen in Simulatortests. Die Firma FRIATEC hat nie Kugelköpfe aus Zirkonoxidkeramik in den Verkehr gebracht, nur Köpfe und Pfannen aus Aluminiumoxidkeramik. Das Pfannendesign wird seit längerer Zeit nicht mehr verwendet, die Produktion ist eingestellt worden.

Die heute allgemein eingesetzte Zirkonoxidkeramik ist ein (metastabiles) Material vom Typ Y-TZP, eine mit **Y**ttrioumoxid stabilisierte **p**olykristalline **Z**irkonoxidkeramik in **t**etragonal Phase. Die tetragonale Phase ist eigentlich nur bei Temperaturen oberhalb ca. 1200°C stabil. Die Phasenumwandlung in die stabile monokline Tieftemperaturphase kann durch Druck, Erhitzung oder Wasser ausgelöst werden. Druck liegt beim Schleifen der Funktionsflächen vor, Erhitzung durch Reibung z. B. bei der Hartbearbeitung und sicherlich in der Gleitpaarung, wenn der Schmierfilm abreißt. Wasser bewirkt Spannungsrißkorrosion. Mit Wasser kommen die Kugelköpfe beim Waschen und eventuell beim Sterilisieren mit Dampf in Kontakt. Die amerikanische Zulassungsbehörde Food and Drug Administration (FDA) hat deshalb das Dampfsterilisieren von Zirkonoxid verboten (16). Neben einer Vorschädigung vor der Implantation ist bei Y-TZP Keramiken auch ein Schädigungsprozeß im Einsatz denkbar, wenn man davon ausgeht, daß im Gelenk in der Reibungszone lokal hohe Temperaturen auftreten können. Im Gegensatz zum weitgehend inerten Aluminiomoxid kann nämlich bei Y-TZP in wässrigen Medien unter erhöhten Temperaturen eine Yttriumverarmung in oberflächennahen Bereichen auftreten, welche dann zu einer lokalen Destabilisierung der tetragonalen Phase führt (tetragonal-monoklinen Umwandlung). Die hiermit verknüpfte Volumenexpansion kann zu Oberflächenschädigungen führen, die bei Belastung einen erhöhten Verschleiß zur Folge haben.

Die gefundenen lokalen Oberflächendefekte und geometrischen Abweichungen lassen die Entstehung von Betriebsgeräuschen durchaus realistisch erscheinen. Eindeutig sind die Toleranzen von Kugelkopf und Pfanne nicht ausreichend abgestimmt, was nicht verwundert, da die Komponenten von zwei Herstellern sind, die wahrscheinlich nie eine Abstimmung über die Toleranzen vereinbart hatten. Die bereits nach 3 Jahren aufgetretenen Verschleißerscheinungen wären bei einer nicht erfolgten Revision höchstwahrscheinlich weiter fortgeschritten und hätten dann später aus anderen Gründen als der Lärmbelästigung zur Folgeoperation geführt.

Dieser Fall macht deutlich, welche negativen Folgen Keramikpaarungen haben können, bei denen die Sphärizität der Artikulationsflächen und das Spiel (der Unterschied der Durchmesser von Kopf und Pfanne) nicht richtig abgestimmt wurden: ein zu geringes Spiel führt zu hoher Reibung, weil die Synovia nicht in den Spalt eindringen kann; ein zu hohes Spiel führt zu extrem hoher Hertz'scher Pressung, die bei Keramik nur durch Bruch, nie durch Verformung aufgelöst werden kann. Unrundheit führt ebenfalls zu extrem hoher lokaler Hertz'scher Pressung.

Schlußfolgerung

Nach heutiger Auslegung sind Komponenten unterschiedlicher Hersteller (und zwar nicht nur für die hier diskutierte Hart/Hart-Gleitpaarung) nicht zugelassen (17), da es weder eine Normung für die Geometrie der einzelnen Komponenten noch ausreichend Absprachen zwischen den verschiedenen Herstellern gibt. Die hier untersuchte Gleitpaarung Aluminiumoxid/Zirkonoxid wurde sicher nie im Sinne der EU-Richtlinien oder der FDA zugelassen.

Der Chirurg, der die Primäroperation durchgeführt hat, ist zum Opfer eines Mißverständnisses geworden, verursacht durch die nicht unübliche unpräzise Nomenklatur: anstatt den von ihm sicher gewünschten positiven Abriebseigenschaften einer „Keramik/Keramik-Hartpaarung" begab er sich in den problematischen Bereich einer Aluminiumoxidkeramik/Zirkonoxidkeramik-Paarung. Der Operator sollte beachten, daß er nur Komponenten kombinieren darf, die dafür zugelassen sind. Im allgemeinen enthält der Beipackzettel diese Informationen. Der sichere Grundsatz lautet: Never mix and match.

Dieses Fallbeispiel dient hoffentlich dazu, in Zukunft derartige Fehler zu vermeiden und die Chirurgen zu motivieren, im Zweifel bei den Herstellern nachzufragen.

Literatur

1 Saikko, V, Pfaff, H.-G., Low wear and friction in alumina/alumina total hip joints: A hip simulator study Acta Orthop. Scand. 69 (1998), 443–448.
2 Refior, J.J., Plitz, W., Walter, A., Ex-vivo and in-vitro analysis of the alumina/alumina bearing system for hip joint prostheses, Bioceramics, 10, 1997, 127–130.
3 Taylor, S. K., Serekian, P. Manley, M., Wear Performance of a Contemporary Alumina/Alumina Bearing Couple Under Hip Joint Simulation. 44th Annual Meeting, Orthopaedic Research Society, March 15–19, New Orleans, Louisiana, USA, 1998, 51–9.
4 Henßge, E .J., Bos, I., Willmann, G., Al_2O_3 against Al_2O_3 combination in hip endoprotheses. Histologic investigations with semiquantitative grading of revision and autopsy cases and abrasion measures. J. Mat. Sci. Mat. in Medicine, 5, 1994, 657–661.

5 Walter, A., On the Material and the Tribology of Alumina-Alumina Coupling for Hip Joint Protheses. Clinical Orthopedics and Related Research 282, 1992, 31–46.
6 Puhl, W. (ed.) Performance of the Wear Couple BIOLOX forte in Hip Arthroplasty. Enke Verlag, Stuttgart 1997.
7 Puhl, W. (ed.) Bioceramics in Orthopaedics – New Applications. Enke Verlag, Stuttgart 1998.
8 Willmann, G., Ceramics for Total Hip Replacement – What a Surgeon Should Know. Orthopaedics 21, 1998, 173–177.
9 Willmann, G., Früh, H. J., Pfaff, H. G., Wear Characteristics of Sliding Pairs of Zirconia (Y-TZP) for Hip Endoprotheses, Biomaterials 17, 1996, 2157–2162.
10 Früh, H.J., Willmann, G., Pfaff, H.G., Wear Characteristic of Ceramic-on-ceramic for Hip Endoprotheses, Biomaterials 18, 1997, 873–876.
11 ISO 6474, Implants for surgery – Ceramic materials based on alumina. ISO 6474 1st ed., 1981.
12 ISO 6474, Implants for surgery – Ceramic materials based on high purity alumina. ISO 6474, 2nd ed., 1994.
13 Clarke, I. ,Willmann, G., Structural Ceramics in Orthopedics. In: Cameron, H.U. (ed.) „Bone Implant Interface", Mosby Pub., St. Louis, 1994, 203–252.
14 Sauer, W.L., Anthony, M.E., Predicting the Clinical Wear Performance of Orthopaedic Bearing Surfaces. In: Jacobs, J. J., Th. L. Craig (eds.): Alternative Bearing Surfaces in Total Joint Replacement STP 1346, ASTM, West Conshohocke, PA, USA 1998, Page 1–29.
15 Villermaux, F., Blaise, L., Drouin, J.M., Cales, B., Ceramic – ceramic Bearing Systems for THP with Zirconia Heads, Bioceramics 11, 1998, 73–76
16 Food and Drug Administration, Steam Re-Sterilization Causes Deterioration of Zirconia Ceramic Heads of Total Hip Protheses, **http://www.fda.gov/cdrh/steamst.html**, May 21, 1997, (FDA) Food and Drug Administration, Washington D.C. USA, 1997.
17 Willmann, G., Keramische Pfannen für Hüftendoprothesen, Teil 4: Never mix and match, Biomed. Technik 43, 1998, 184–186.

4 CeramTec Award

4.1 CeramTec Awards for Studies in the Field of Bioceramics 1996–1999

At the occasion of the International Symposiums in Stuttgart, Germany CeramTec (formerly CERASIV) has awarded a prize for outstanding studies with regard to the problems of wear in total joint replacment. This prize shall be awarded to young surgeons, engineers, or scientists who published or submitted as a publication or thesis these research results in the field of wear couple in orthopaedics.

The winner of the CeramTec Award 1999 is Florence Prudhommeaux (Paris)

with the paper „**Analysis of Alumina – alumina Hip Prostheses Wear Behavior after 10 Years of Implantation**"

The paper is submitted to Clin. Orthop. Rel Res.
For the abstract see page 105.

The winner of the prices of 1996 to 1998 had been:

1998: Lu, Z., H. McKellop
With the paper „Frictional heating of bearing materials tested in a hip joint simulator" Proc. Instn. mech. Engrs 211 Part H (1997) 101–108

1997: Th. Lindenfeld
„In vivo Verschleiß der Gleitpaarungen Keramik – Polyethylen gegen Metall – Polyethylen" [In vivo wear of the wear couples ceramics-on-poly ethylene and metal-on-polyethylene]
Orthopäde 26 (1997) 129–34

1996: E. Fritsch
„Biocompatibility of Alumina – Ceramic in Total Hip Replacement. Macroscopic – and Microscopic Findings on capsular Tissues after Long-term Implantation"
pages 12–17 in: W. Puhl (ed.) „Die Keramikpaarung BIOLOX in der Hüftendoprothetik"
[The ceramic Wear Couple BIOLOX in Total Hip Replacement]
Proc. 1st Int. Symposium in Stuttgart, March 23, 1996
Enke Verlag Stuttgart 1996

4.2 Analysis of Alumina-Alumina Hip Prostheses Wear Behavior after 10 Years of Implantation[*]

F. Prudhommeaux, J. Nevelos, M. Amadouche, C. Doyle, A. Meunier, L. Sedel

Abstract

The aim of this study was to investigate the surface topography of 11 Al_2O_3-Al_2O_3 hip prostheses retrieved for aseptic loosening, after a mean implantation time of 11 years. Macroscopic wear features were assessed by measuring dimensions' changes, using a coordinate measuring machine (CMM) and microscopic wear features were evaluated by Talysurf analysis. Scanning electron microscopy (SEM) was used to look at the alumina microstructure after thermal etching. Clinical as well as roentgenographic data were reviewed by an independent party.

Components were classified into 3 groups according to their visual wear patterns and characterized as a function of wear magnitude.

„Low wear" (n = 4) with no sign of wear as confirmed by Ra values below 0.05 μm; „Stripe wear" (n = 5) with a visible oblong worn area on heads and characterized by penetration rates below 10 μm/yr; and „Severe wear" (n = 2) with a visible loss of material on both components, showing Rt values up to 4 μm and maximum penetrations higher than 150 μm. Alumina quality assessed by grain size measurements and porosity percentages appeared to improve progressively during the 1977–1988 period of interest. This resulted in a correlated decrease of the microscopic wear magnitude. However, on a macroscopic scale, penetration rates were emphasized by a combination of unfavorable factors responsible for increasing the load (patients weight, young age, and male gender) the joint was submitted or impairing the load's distribution over the component surfaces (large grain size, non optimal initial cup inclination, and occurrence of cup migration and/or tilting).

As a conclusion, the use of alumina-alumina bearing surfaces is safe, but its use should not be advocated to patients without a risk evaluation inquiry.

KEY WORDS: Total Joint Arthroplasty; Alumina; Retrieved implants; Wear.

---

[*] Paper submitted to Clin. Orthop. Rel. Res.

5 Important References

5.1 A Bibliography of Published Literature on Bioceramics for THR: 1st Update

G. Willmann

1 Bioceramics in Orthopaedics

Since the 1970's when first it was realized that the properties of alumina ceramics could be exploited to provide better implants for orthopaedic applications, the field has expanded enormously. Initial applications depended on the fact that alumina ceramics were bioinert and provided wear characteristics suitable for bearing surfaces.

Resultant orthopaedic use has enjoyed more than 25 years' clinical success, e.g. BIOLOX®forte alumina femoral heads, sockets, and acetabular liners for total hip replacement. About 10 years ago zirconia was approved for use as femoral ball heads articulating against polyethylene cups.

The bioactive hydroxyaptite offers attractive tissue reactions. It is well established as coating on metal implants to enhance osseointegration. Hydroxyapatite (HA) is used for bone grafting, too.

The bioceramics mentioned are commercially used in Northern America, Japan, Australia, and Europe. There are lots of publications, reviews, and books about application of bioceramics. A bibliography has been published by G. Willmann.[1]

This bibliography was updated compiling latest papers, reviews, books and standards that became known to the author in 1998.

In 1999 there is the 25th anniversary of clinical use of BIOLOX®forte in total hip replacement. Some pioneer papers have been included.

2 Reviews, Proceedings, and Books

Black J, Jacobs JJ (1998) Materials for Alternate bearings: Biological Considerations. Seminars of Arthroplasty 9: 157–164

Black J, Hastings G (ed) (1998) Handbook of Biomaterial Properties. Chapman & Hall, London

CeramTec AG (1998) BIOLOX®'forte and BIOLOX®zirconia: Technical data and product range – hip replacement. Brochure CeramTec AG Plochingen

Claes LA, Ignatius A (ed) (1998) Biodegradierbare Implantate und Materialien. Hefte zur Unfallchirurgie Heft 265, Springer Verlag, Berlin, Heidelberg, New York

Cuckler JM (1998) Ceramic – Polyethylene Articulation: Rationale, Indication, and Results. Seminars of Arthroplasty 9: 176–180

Dalla Pria P (1997) The ceramic–ceramic coupling in hip prosthesis. Brochure by Lima, Italy

Garino JP (1999) Total Hip Replacement: The Next Generation. Seminars of Arthroplasty 9: 98–104

Garino J, (1998) Ceramic on Ceramic and Alternate Bearing Surfaces in Total Hip Replacement. Proc 1st Ann Symp in Philadelphia (Proc will be published in CORR)

Havelin L (1995) Hip Arthroplasty in Norway 1987–1994 – The Norwegian Arthroplasty Register. Dep Surgery and Section of Medical Informatics and Statistics, University of Bergen, Bergen, Norway

Heisel J, Jerosch J (ed) (1998) Das künstliche Hüftgelenk Wichtige Fragen und Antworten. CeramTec Informationsschrift, Plochingen, Germany

Hench LL (1998) Bioceramics. J Amer Ceram Soc 81: 1705–28

Heros R, Willmann G (1998) Ceramics in Total Hip Arthroplasty: History, Mechanical Properties, Clinical results and Current Manufacturing State of the Art. Seminars of Arthroplasty 9: 114–122

Jerosch J, Heisel J (1997) Leben mit einem künstlichen Gelenk – Endoprothesenschule. DTV Ratgeber, München

La Berge M, (1998) Wear. In: Black J, Hastings G (ed) Handbook of Biomaterial Properties. Chapman & Hall, London, 364–405

LeGeros, RZ, LeGeros JP (eds) (1998) Bioceramics 11. World Sci Publ Co, Singapore, New Jersey, London, HongKong

Li J, Hastings G (ed) (1998) Oxide bioceramics: inert ceramic materials in medicine and dentistry. In: Black J, Hastings G (ed) Handbook of Biomaterial Properties. Chapman & Hall, London, 340–354

---

[1] Willmann G (1998): A Bibliography of Published Literature on Bioceramics for THR. In: Puhl W (ed) Bioceramics in Orthopaedics – New Applications. ENKE Verlag Stuttgart, 132–136

Li S, Furman BD, Gillis AM (1998) Polyethylene: can it be Made Better? Seminars of Arthroplasty 9: 105–113

Orthopaedics today (ed) (1998) 1st Annual Consumers Guide to Total Hip Systems 1998. Orthopaedics today Int 1: No 6, 17–26

Parr JE, Mayor MB, Marlowe DE (ed) (1997) Modularity of Orthopedic Implants. ASTM ST 1301 American Soc for Testing and Materials, Philadelphia, PA, USA

Puhl W (ed) (1998) Bioceramics in Orthopaedics – New Applications. Enke Verlag, Stuttgart

Samntavirta S, Konttinen YT, Lappalainen R, Anttila A, Goodman SB, Lind M, (1998). Materials in total joint replacement. Current Orthopaedics 12: 51–57

Sedel L, Rey Ch (eds) (1997) Bioceramics 10. Pergamon, Elsevier Sci. Ltd., Oxford

Sedel L, Cabanela ME (ed) (1998) Hip Surgery – Materials and Developments. Martin Dunitz, London

Schnettler R, Markgraf E (eds) (1998) Knochenersatzmaterialien und Wachstumsfaktoren. Georg Thieme Verlag, Stuttgart, New York

Sedel L, Nizard R, Bizot P, Meunier A (1998) Perspective on a 20-Year Experience with Ceramic-on-ceramic Articulation in Total Hip Replacement. Seminars of Arthroplasty 9: 123–134

Stegmaier A (1997) Konstruktive Entwicklung von keramischen Pfannen für Hüft-Endoprothesen. Diplomarbeit Universität Stuttgart, Inst f Biomed Technik

The Association of Bone & Joint Surgeons (1998) Orthopaedic Device Reference 1st ed. Breckenridge Publ Comp Breckenridge, Colorado, USA

Willmann G (1998) Hip-Joint Replacement: Still a Challenge to Orthopaedists, Tribologists and Designers. In: Bartz WJ (ed) Industrial and Automotive Lubrication. Proc 11th Int Coll 13–15 Jan 1998, Technische Akademie Ostfildern, Germany, 7–21

3 Government Regulations and Standards

ASTM F 1609-95 (1995) Standard Specification for Calcium Phosphate Coatings for Implantable Materials. American Soc for Testing and Materials, Philadelphia, PA, USA

ASTM F 1044-95 (1995) Standard Test method for Shear Testing of Porous Metal Coatings. American Soc. for Testing and Materials, Philadelphia, PA, USA

ASTM F 1088-87 (1987) Standard Specification for Beta-Tricalcium Phosphate for Surgical Implantions. American Soc for Testing and Materials, Philadelphia, PA, USA

Castro FP, Chimento G, Munn BG, Levy RS, Tiomon S, Barrack RL (1997) An Analysis of Food and Drug Administration medical Device Reports Relating to Total Joint Components. J Arthroplasty 12: 765–770

DIN EN 12563 (1996) Implantate für den Gelenkersatz – Spezielle Anforderungen an Implantate für den Hüftgelenkersatz. DIN EN 12563, Dez 1996

Food and Drug Administration (1997) Steam Re-Sterilization Causes Deterioration of Zirconia Ceramic Heads of Total Hip Protheses. http://www.fda.gov/cdrh/steamst.html, May 21, 1997, Food and Drug Administration, Washington, D C USA

ISO/CD 14242 (1997) Implants for surgery – Wear of total hip joint Prostheses.

ISO/CD 14879, ISO/CD 14243 (1997) Implants for surgery – Wear of total knee joint Prostheses.

4 Wear Couples for hip joints

Anderson P (1992) Water – lubricated pin-on-disc test with ceramics. Wear 154: 37–47

Bädorf D, Willmann G (1998) Polyethylen in der Totalendoprothetik – Eine Sackgasse für Dauerimplantates? Biomed Technik 43: 151

Bergmann G, Graichen F, Rohlmann A (1999) Reibungsbedingte Erwärmung von Hüftendoprothesen. Abstract Dt Ges f Biomechanik Ulm 26./27. Febr. 99

Boehler M, Krismer M, Mayr G, Mühlbauer M, Salzer M (1998) Migration Measurement of Cementless Acetabular Components: Value of Clinical and Radiographic Data. Orthopaedics 21: 897–900

Blömer W (1997) Biomechanical aspects of modular inlay fixation. Hip Int 7: 110–120

Chevalier J, Drouin JM, Cales B (1997) Low temperature aging behaviour of zirconia hip joint heads. Bioceramics 10: 135–138

Früh HJ, Willmann G (1998) Tribological Investigations of the Wear Couple Alumina and CFRP for Total Hip Replacement. Biomaterials 19: 1145–1150

Clarke IC, Good V, Anissan L, Gustafson A (1997) Charnley wear model for validation of hip simulator – ball diameter vs polytetrafluoroethylene and polyethylene wear. Proc Instn Mech Engrs 211 Part H: 25–36

Davidson JA (1993) Characteristics of metal and ceramic total hip bearing surfaces and their effect on long-term ultra high molecular weight polyethylene wear. Clin Orthop Rel Res 294: 361–378

Dowson D (1998) A comparative study of the performance of metallic and ceramic femoral head component in total replacement hip joints. Wear 190: 171–183

Geldbach J (1999) Keramik in der Hüftendoprothetik – Eine multizentrische Studie zur Keramiksicherheit (Überlegungen zur Keramiksicherheit aufgrund multizentrisch-erhobener Daten). Dissertation Medizinische Fakultät Heidelberg der Ruprecht-Karls-Universität

Good V, Clarke IC, Anissan L (1996) Water and Bovine Serum Lubrication Compared in Simulator PTFE / CoCr Wear Model. J Biomed Mat Res (Appl Biomaterials) 33: 275–283

Gotman I (1997) Characteristics of metals used in implants. J Endourology 11: 383–389

Hamadouche M, Bizot P, Nizard RS, Sedel L (1997) Hybrid alumina- alumina hip replacement: A survivorship analysis and results at a minimal five year follow-up. Bioceramics 10: 131–134

Heimann RB, Willmann G (1997) Irridation induced colour changes in medical grade Y-TZP ceramics. Brit Ceram Trans 97: 185–188

Hirakawa K, Bauer TW, Hashimoto Y, Stulberg BN, Wilde AH, Secic (1997) Effect of femoral head diameter on

tissue concentration of wear debris. J Biomed Mater Res 36: 529-535
Jasty M, Bragdon C, Lee K, Hanson A, Harris W (1997) Surface Damage to Cobalt – Chrome Femoral Head Prostheses. J Bone Joint Surg (Br) 76 B: 73-77
Kusaba A, Kuroki Y (1997) Femoral Component Wear in Retrieved Hip Prostheses. J Bone Joint Surgery 79 B: 331-336
Lancester JG, Dowson D, Isaac GH, Fisher J (1997) The wear of ultra-high molecular weight polyethylene sliding on metallic and ceramic counterfaces representative of curent femoral surfaces in joint replacement. J Eng in Medicine 211:17-24
Learmonth ID, Cunningham JL (1997) Factors contributing to the wear of polyethylene in clinical practice. J Eng in Medicine 211: 49-57
Minakawa H, Ignham E, Tipper JL, Stone M, Wroblewski BM, Fisher J (1997) Why Do Ceramic Femoral Heads Produe Lower Polyethylene Wear in Artificial Joints? In: Proc Int Conf on New Frontiers in Biomechanical Engineering, Tokyo, Japan, July 18/19, 331-334
Pfaff HG, Willmann G (1998) Stability of Y-TZP Zirconia. In: Puhl W (ed) Bioceramics in Orthopaedics – New Applications. Enke Verlag, Stuttgart, 29-31
Piconi C, Burger W, Richter HG, Cittadini A, Maccauro G, Covaccio V, Bruzzese N, Ricci G, Marmo E (1998) Y-TZP ceramics for artificial joint replacements Biomaterials 19: 1489-1494
Prudhommeaux F, Nevelos J, Doyle, Meunier A, Sedel L (1998) Analysis of Wear Behavior of Alumina – alumina Hip Prostheses after 10 Years of Implantation. Bioceramics 11: 621-624
Quack G, Krahl H, Asmuth T, a d Fünten K, Willmann G, Grundei H (1997) Keramik-Keramik-Gleitpaarung als Perspektive bei metallspongiösem modularem Pfannensystem auf der Grundlage 9jähriger Erfahrung. Orthop Praxis 33: 577-587
Refior J, Plitz W, Walter A (1997) Ex vivo and in vitro analysis of the alumina / alumina bearing system for hip joint prostheses. Bioceramics 10: 127-130
Semlitsch M, Willert HG (1997) Clinical wear behaviour of ultra-high molecular weight polyethylene paired with metal and ceramic ball heads in comparison to metal-on-metal pairings of hip joint replacement. J Eng in Medicine 211:73-88
Sugano N, Nishii T, Nakata K, Masuhara K, Takaokoa K (1995) Polyethylene Sockets and Alumina Ceramics Heads in Cemented Total Hip Arthroplasty – A Ten-year Study. J Bone Joint Surgery 77-B: 548-556
Villermaux F, Blaise L, Drouin JM, Cales B (1998) Ceramic – ceramic Bearing Systems for THP with Zirconia Heads. Bioceramics 11: 73-76
Willmann G (1997) Keramische Pfannen für Hüftendoprothesen Teil 3: Zum Problem der Osteointegration monolithischer Pfannen. Biomed Technik 42: 256-263
Willmann G, Brodbeck A (1998) Investigation of 87 Retrieved Ceramic Femoral Heads. Bioceramics 11: 625-628
Willmann G, von Chamier W (1998) The Improvements of the Materials Properties of BIOLOX Offer Benefits for THR. Bioceramics 11: 649-652
Willmann G, Kramer U (1998) Keramische Pfannen für Hüftendoprothesen Teil 5: Konzeptionelle Überlegungen. Biomed Technik 43: 342-349
Willmann G (1998) Überlebenswahrscheinlichkeit und Sicherheit von keramischen Kugelköpfen für Hüftendoprothesen. Mat u wiss Werkstofftechnik 29: 595-604

5 Some Pioneer Papers about Ceramics for THR

Boutin PM (1971) L'alumine et son utilisation en chirurgie de la hanche. Presse Méd. 79: 14
Boutin PM (1972) Arthroplastic totale de hanche par prothese en alumine fritte. Rev Chi Orthop 58: 229 246
von Andrian-Werburg H, Griss P, Krempien B, Heimke G (1973) Klinische Problematik und experimentell morphologische Befunde bei der Verwendung keramischer Werkstoffe in der Orthopädie und Unfallchirurgie. Z Orthopädie 111: 577-579
Mittelmeier H (1975) Selbsthaftende Keramik – Metall – Verbund – Endoprothese. Med Orthop Technik 95: 152-159
Oonishi H, Igaki H, Takayama Y (1989) Comparision of Wear of UHMW Polyethylene Sliding against Metal and Alumina in Total Hip Protheses. Bioceramics 1: 272-277
Oonishi H (1992) Bioceramics in Orthopaedic Surgery – Our Clinical Experience. Bioceramics 3: 31-42
Salzer M, Zweymüller K, Locke H, Plenk H jr, Punzet G (1975) Biokeramische Endoprothesen. Med Orthop Technik 95: 40-45
Salzer M, Zweymüller K, Locke H, Plenk H jr, Punzet G (1975) Erste Erfahrungen mit einer Hüfttotalendoprothese aus Biokeramik. Med Orthop Technik 95: 162-164

6 Bioactive Ceramics

Baroud, G, Willmann G, Kreißig R (1998) A Numerical Consideration of Hip Prostheses Coating on the Post – operative Biomechanical State of the Femur. Bioceramics 11: 611-615
Kinner B, Willmann G, Storz S, Kinner J (1997) Bringt die Hydroxylapatit – Beschichtung makroporöser Hüftendoprothesen eine Verbesserung? In: Oestern HJ, Rehm KE (eds) Hefte Unfallchirurgie, 61 Jahrestagung Dt Ges Unfallchirurgie, Springer Verlag, Berlin, 351-356
Kinner B, Willmann G, Storz S, Kinner J (1998) Erfahrungen mit einer Hydroxylapatit-beschichteten, makroporös strukturierten Hüftendoprothese. Z Orthop 136: im Druck
Lintner F, Huber M, Böhm G, Scholz, Attems J (1998) Histologisch-morphometrische Untersuchungen zum Zustand der HA-Beschichtung nach mehrjähriger Implantation. Osteologie 7: 92-104
Krüger, TH, Reichel H, Bernstein A, Hein W (1997) Die Hydroxylapatitbeschichtung in der zementfreien Endoprothetik – Ergebnisse einer histologischen Studie. Osteosynthese Int 5: 54-59

Moroni A, Faldidi C, Heikkila J, Larson ST, Magyar G, Stea S, Zhou J, Gianna S (1998) Clinical Study on Hydroxyapatite Coated External Fixations Pins. Bioceramics 11: 617–620

Ogiso M, Yamashita Y, Matsumoto T (1998) The Process of Physical Weakening and Dissolution of the HA-Coated Implant in Bone and Soft Tissue. J Dent Res 77: 1426–1434

Rueger JM (1998) Knochenersatzmittel. Orthopädie 27: 72–79

Rueger JM (1998) Synthetische resorbierbare Materialien: Eine Alternative zum Transplantat? In: Claes LA, Ignatius A (ed) (1998) Biodegradierbare Implantate und Materialien. Hefte zur Unfallchirurgie Heft 265, Springer Verlag, Berlin, Heidelberg, New York, 261–269